MASTERING
NEUROSCIENCE
A LABORATORY GUIDE

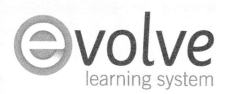

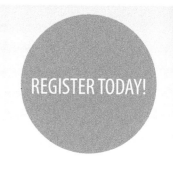

REGISTER TODAY!

To access your Student Resources, visit:

http://evolve.elsevier.com/Schaaf/neuroscience/

Evolve Instructor Resources for Schaaf/Zapletal's Mastering Neuroscience: A Laboratory Guide offers the following features:

- **Instructor Lab Manual**
  Answers to the exercises in the student lab manual.

- **Pathway Figure**
  Full-page copy that can be laminated and handed out to students.

- **Sample Syllabus**
  Guide for course structure and pace.

NOTE: Instructors should check with their Elsevier sales representative for further information.

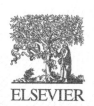

ELSEVIER

MASTERING
NEUROSCIENCE
A LABORATORY GUIDE

Roseann C. Schaaf, PhD, OTR/L, FAOTA

Associate Professor, Vice Chairman
Department of Occupational Therapy
School of Health Professions
Thomas Jefferson University
Philadelphia, Pennsylvania

Audrey L. Zapletal, MS, OTR/L

Instructor
Department of Occupational Therapy
School of Health Professions
Thomas Jefferson University
Philadelphia, Pennsylvania

With 74 illustrations

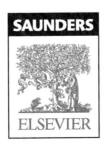

SAUNDERS

ELSEVIER

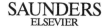

11830 Westline Industrial Drive
St. Louis, Missouri 63146

MASTERING NEUROSCIENCE
Copyright © 2010 by Saunders, an imprint of Elsevier Inc.

ISBN: 978-1-4160-6222-6

Notice

Knowledge and best practice in this field are constantly changing. As new research and experience broaden our knowledge, changes in practice, treatment and drug therapy may become necessary or appropriate. Readers are advised to check the most current information provided (i) on procedures featured or (ii) by the manufacturer of each product to be administered, to verify the recommended dose or formula, the method and duration of administration, and contraindications. It is the responsibility of the practitioner, relying on their own experience and knowledge of the patient, to make diagnoses, to determine dosages and the best treatment for each individual patient, and to take all appropriate safety precautions. To the fullest extent of the law, neither the Publisher nor the Authors assumes any liability for any injury and/or damage to persons or property arising out of or related to any use of the material contained in this book.

The Publisher

ISBN: 978-1-4160-6222-6

Vice President and Publisher: Linda Duncan
Executive Editor: Kathy Falk
Senior Developmental Editor: Melissa Kuster Deutsch
Editorial Assistant: Lindsay Westbrook
Publishing Services Manager: Catherine Jackson
Project Manager: Jennifer Boudreau
Design Direction: Charlie Siebel
Cover Designer: Charlie Siebel

Printed in the United States of America

Transferred to Digital Printing, 2014

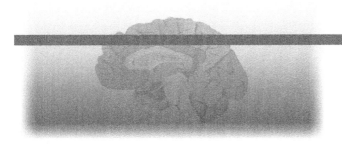

This manual is dedicated to the memory of Dr. Richard Berry, who gave of his time, talents, and wisdom to the occupational therapy program at Thomas Jefferson University, 1983-1999.

Editorial Review Board

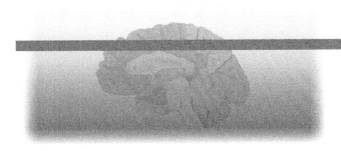

GENERAL INSTRUCTIONS FOR USING LAB MANUAL AND BRAIN SPECIMENS

How to Use This Lab Manual
For maximal benefit, this guide should be used in conjunction with a neuroscience textbook (see our recommendations at the end of this section). It is also helpful to have brain specimens or models in order to have a three dimensional view of these brain structures. If you have access to lab specimens, please refer to the section "How to Handle and Care for Brain Specimens."

Organization of the Lab
This self-guided manual is organized as follows: at the beginning of each lab, clear goals are stated. Specific instructions are provided for the student to complete the lab. Labs 2-5 contain a review section to assist the student's understanding of pertinent, previously learned material. Space is provided for the lab instructor's signature, to indicate that the student has completed the lab prep assignment prior to class. We recommend the first 30 minutes of each lab be dedicated to gathering students in groups of two or three to check lab assignment answers as the lab instructor checks the homework for completion. Afterwards, the lab instructor and students work together to ensure understanding of the lab material and concepts.

Lab Preparation
Prior to lab, students independently complete the lab prep assignment that is provided at the beginning of the lab. The assignment usually consists of completing a review section focused on previously learned material and preparing for the current lab by locating pictures from a variety of textbooks that demonstrate the desired structure(s) and answering questions. Students should expect to spend 3-5 hours preparing for each lab.

Each lab session includes specific instructions to assist you in preparing for it. Your preparations should be completed before you enter the lab to begin a session. Prepare for Labs 1-5, which focus on the identification of brain structures, by using a textbook to locate pictures and then answering questions and case examples. Labs 6-13 involve the neurophysiologic contributions to movement and behavior. You will identify pertinent structures within the nervous system, draw pathways outlining the neural circuits, and answer case stories that illustrate dysfunction in specific areas of the brain. Refer to a textbook for supplementary materials to augment this section. When completing any lab homework, it is helpful to write the page number and the name of the text in the lab book for quick reference during lab and for later study.

Please refer to your syllabus for additional instructions regarding lab preparation assignments.

How to Handle and Care for Brain Specimens
The contents of the specimen container include a whole brain, a hemisected brain, a brainstem with or without cerebellum attached, a spinal cord, brainstem cross sections, and a set of coronal slices. These specimens have been fixed and stored in formalin-like solution. Only the specimen required for immediate use should be removed from the container. The material is extremely susceptible to drying and is easily ruined for further study by the resulting discoloration. A wet paper towel placed around the specimen while you are working will help keep it moist. At the end of each lab, replace the specimens in the container, drape a damp cloth or paper towel over the surface to prevent the specimens from drying, and put the lid *securely* on the container. Clean and dry your trays. Brain tissue is very fragile and will crumble under excess pressure. Avoid damage from too much traction. To prevent punctures, a blunt instrument should be used for demonstrating structures. Be sure to examine other specimens as well as your own in order to appreciate the variability of the material.

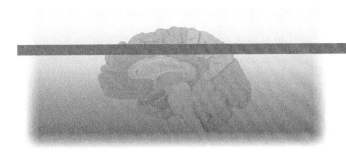

THE FOLLOWING TEXTS ARE RECOMMENDED AS ADJUNCTS TO THE PRIMARY TEXT:

Lundy-Ekman L: *Neuroscience: Fundamentals for Rehabilitation*, ed 3, Philadelphia, 2007, Saunders.

Nolte J: *The Human Brain*, ed 5, Philadelphia, 2002, Mosby.

Haines D: *Neuroanatomy: An Atlas of Structures, Sections, and Systems*, ed 7, Philadelphia, 2008, Lippincott Williams & Wilkins.

Diamond MC, Scheibel AB, Elson LM: *The Human Brain Coloring Book*, New York, 1985, Harper & Row.

Netter F: *Atlas of Human Anatomy*, ed 4, Philadelphia, 2006, Elsevier.

Sidman RL, Sidman M: *Neuroanatomy, A Programmed Text*, vol 1, Boston, 1965, Little, Brown & Co.

Acknowledgments

This manual/workbook was compiled with the help of several people and sources who deserve proper acknowledgement. Dr. Richard Berry, Professor Emeritus, Dept. of Neuropathology, Thomas Jefferson University, Philadelphia, PA, edited, reviewed, and clarified much of the content in the manual. Carolyn M. Scott, MS, LPT, Pennsylvania Hospital Dept. of Physical Therapy, Philadelphia, PA, assisted in the reviewing and editing earlier versions of this manual. Nancy Thomas, MEd, OTR/L, Ithaca, NY, contributed case studies for the spinal cord and brain stem lesion sections of the manual. Teal Benevides, MS, OTR/L, and Heather Schwenk, MS, OTR/L, Thomas Jefferson University, Department of Occupational Therapy, Philadelphia, PA, contributed ideas for lab activities and assisted in the editing of this manual for several years. Their enthusiasm for neuroanatomy and learning is contagious. Finally, and most importantly, we would like to thank our husbands David Schaaf and Ross Berkowitz for their support and encouragement.

Without the generous assistance from these people, this laboratory manual would not have the quality information it contains. Our sincere thanks to each of these persons.

Roseann C. Schaaf
and Audrey L. Zapletal

Contents

Gross Central Nervous System

Gross Central Nervous System

MATERIALS
Brain specimens; brain; ventricular and brainstem models; books, atlas

GOAL

The goal of this lab is to familiarize you with the brain specimens, the various sections, and major divisions and components of the brain, brainstem, and spinal cord.

PREPARATION FOR LAB

Use your textbooks and atlas to find the structures. Indicate on each lab section the page number of the textbook showing photos of the structures in each section. For example, in the "Whole Brain" section, indicate a textbook page number showing the cerebral hemispheres, the longitudinal fissure, the diencephalon, etc. Bring these texts to lab to use as references. During lab, you will locate these structures on the specimens or models.

1. Define the terms and sections:

   a. Sagittal

   b. Coronal/frontal

   c. Horizontal

2. Locate the whole brain specimen and the following structures as shown in Figure 1-1.

Whole Brain

Divisions of the Whole Brain

On the whole brain, note the following divisions and lobes of the brain:

1. Cerebral hemispheres

   a. Longitudinal fissure

2. Diencephalon

3. Brainstem

   a. Medulla

   b. Pons

   c. Midbrain

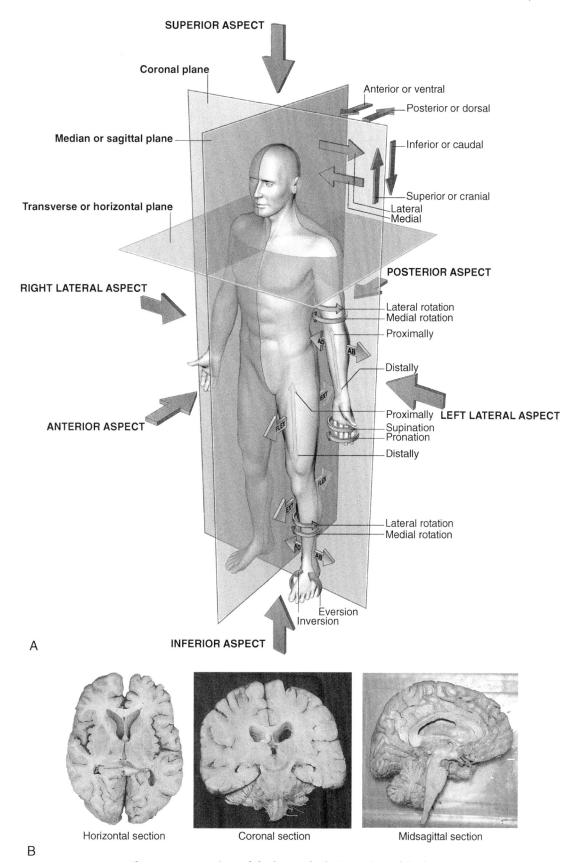

A

SUPERIOR ASPECT

Coronal plane

Anterior or ventral

Posterior or dorsal

Median or sagittal plane

Inferior or caudal

Transverse or horizontal plane

Superior or cranial
Lateral
Medial

POSTERIOR ASPECT

RIGHT LATERAL ASPECT

Lateral rotation
Medial rotation

Proximally

Distally

Proximally   LEFT LATERAL ASPECT
Supination
Pronation

Distally

ANTERIOR ASPECT

Lateral rotation
Medial rotation

Eversion
Inversion

INFERIOR ASPECT

B

Horizontal section   Coronal section   Midsagittal section

Figure 1-1 A, Sections of the human body. **B,** Sections of the brain.

4. Cerebellum

   a. Left and right lobes of the cerebellum

   b. The vermis (midline structure)

5. Meninges: protective coverings of the brain

   a. Dura mater

   b. Arachnoid

   c. Pia mater

Lobes of the Brain

1. Frontal

2. Parietal

3. Temporal

4. Occipital

Sagittal Section of the Brain

1. Note the space of the third, lateral, and fourth ventricles.

2. Find the thalamus, an egg-shaped structure in the diencephalon.

3. Note the corpus callosum, the midline structure that links the right and left hemispheres of the cortex.

4. Identify the medulla, pons, midbrain, and diencephalon on the sagittal section.

CORONAL SECTIONS: VENTRICULAR SYSTEM

Lateral ventricle: Comment on how the lateral ventricle changes shape moving from the frontal lobe to the occipital lobe.

Spinal Cord Anatomy

On the whole spinal cord, locate the following:

1. Spinal cord

2. Spinal nerves

3. The spinal nerves are composed of _____ and _____ roots.

4. Dura mater of the spinal cord

Sulci, Gyri and Fissures

Strip away as little of the meninges as possible (these cover the outer surfaces of the cortex) to examine the various sulci, gyri, and fissures.

1. What is the difference between sulci, gyri, and fissures?

2. Locate each of the following structures and write the general location of the structure listed below.

Structure	Location
Central sulcus (of Rolando)	
Precentral gyrus	
Postcentral gyrus	
Lateral fissure (sulcus of Sylvius)	
Medial longitudinal fissure	

Locate the parahippocampal gyrus and cingulate gyrus. You may need to gently lift the cerebellum to find the parahippocampal gyrus. They will be examined in the sagittal section as well.

3. The parahippocampal gyrus and cingulate gyrus are located in the _____ lobe.

   a. Define the general function of this lobe.

4. The parahippocampal gyrus ends in what structure?

Locate the corpus callosum by gently separating the cerebral hemispheres at the medial longitudinal fissure.

5. What is the function of the corpus callosum?

Inferior Surface of the Whole Brain

These are important landmarks that orient you to the anterior surface of the brainstem and/or the inferior surface of the brain. On the inferior surface of the brain, identify the following structures:

1. The medulla

2. The pons

3. The mammillary bodies

4. The optic chiasm

5. The infundibular stalk

Structures of the Brain

1. Label the structures identified on Figure 1-2.

A. _____

B. _____

C. _____

D. _____

E. _____

F. _____

G. _____

H. _____

I. _____

J. _____

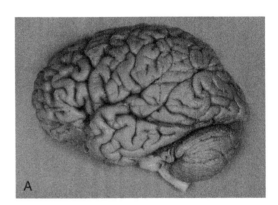

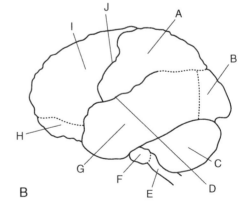

Figure 1-2 Lobes and fissures of the brain (lateral view).

2. Label the structures identified on Figure 1-3.

A. _____

B. _____

C. _____

D. _____

E. _____

F. _____

G. _____

H. _____

I. _____

J. _____

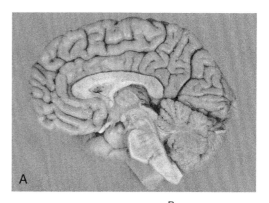

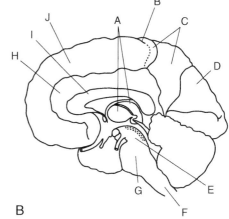

Figure 1-3 Structures of the brain (sagittal view).

3. Label the structures identified on Figure 1-4.

   A. _____

   B. _____

   C. _____

   D. _____

   E. _____

   F. _____

   G. _____

   H. _____

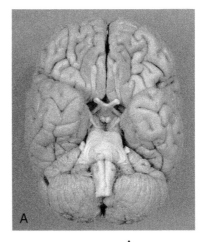

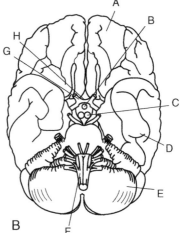

Figure 1-4 Structures of the brain (inferior view).

2. Label the structures identified on Figure 1-3.

A. _____

B. _____

C. _____

D. _____

E. _____

F. _____

G. _____

H. _____

I. _____

J. _____

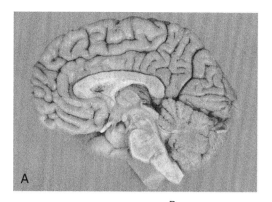

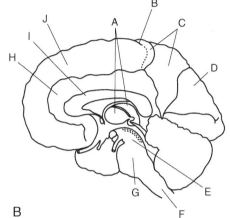

Figure 1-3 Structures of the brain (sagittal view).

3. Label the structures identified on Figure 1-4.

A. _____

B. _____

C. _____

D. _____

E. _____

F. _____

G. _____

H. _____

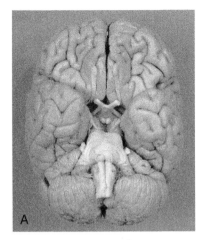

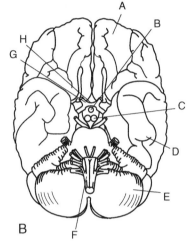

Figure 1-4 Structures of the brain (inferior view).

2

Brainstem and Sagittal Sections

Brainstem and Sagittal Sections

MATERIALS
Brain specimens, ventricular and brainstem models, books, atlas

GOAL

In this lab, you will study the external structures and function of the brain and brainstem and then begin to investigate the internal structures on the sagittal section.

PREPARATION FOR LAB

It takes 3 to 5 hours to prepare for this lab.

1. Complete the review of Lab 1 on the following page. Most of the material has been covered in the introductory lab. Please reference your findings with page numbers. This will help you complete the lab in a timely fashion.

2. Use your textbooks and atlas as a reference. Indicate on each lab section the page number of the textbook showing photos of the structures in each section. Bring these texts to the lab to use as references. You may use the pictures in this lab manual to help you initially identify the structures on the specimen and in other texts.

3. Complete at least 25% of the picture labeling activity.

Your lab instructor will check that you have prepared for the lab and will sign below.

Signature of Lab Instructor

REVIEW OF LAB 1

The diencephalon is not visible on the whole brain because it is hidden by the cerebral hemispheres.
The divisions of the diencephalon will be identified on the sagittal section where they are most visible.

1. What are the structures of the diencephalon?

2. What structure does the infundibular stalk hold?

3. Note the relationship of the optic chiasm and the infundibulum to the diencephalic structures.

4. Gyri and fissures

   a. Name the fissure that separates the two cerebral hemispheres.

   b. Name the structure where conscious motor information originates.

   c. Name the structure that separates the frontal, parietal, and temporal lobes.

LAB 2

Begin this lab by reviewing the whole brain on all surfaces. When you have a general feel for the whole brain and brainstem, study the sagittal section: pay particular attention to the structures you studied on the whole brain and brainstem and relate their appearance to that on the sagittal section.

Brainstem

The brainstem includes the medulla oblongata, the pons, and the midbrain.

1. Label the structures identified on Figure 2-1.

   A. _____

   B. _____

   C. _____

   D. _____

   E. _____

   F. _____

   G. _____

   H. _____

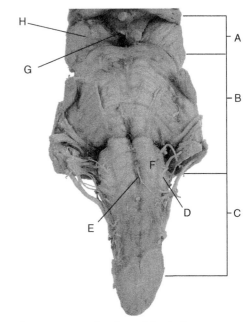

Figure 2-1 Anterior view of the brainstem.

2. Label the structures identified on Figure 2-2.

   A. _____

   B. _____

   C. _____

   D. _____

   E. _____

   F. _____

   G. _____

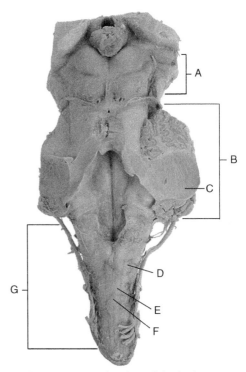

Figure 2-2 Posterior view of the brainstem.

Locate the following structures on the whole brain (when visible), the brainstem models, and then on the sagittal sections. Orient yourself to the ventral and dorsal brainstem by noting which structures are landmarks on each view.

Medulla

Note the rostral and caudal boundaries of the medulla and locate the following structures:

1. Pyramids

2. Anterior median sulcus

3. Fibers of the pyramidal decussation (if visible)

    a. What is the significance of the pyramidal decussation fibers?

4. The inferior olives

5. The dorsal medial sulcus (posterior median sulcus)

6. The fasciculus gracilis and its termination in the nucleus gracilis (posterior aspect)

    a. What types of information are these structures carrying?

7. The fasciculus cuneatus and its termination in the nucleus cuneatus (posterior aspect)

    a. What types of information are these structures carrying?

8. The inferior cerebellar peduncle

    a. This structure is mainly carrying fibers from the _____ to the _____.

Pons

1. Note the rostral and caudal (ventral and dorsal) boundaries of the pons and the ventral and dorsal surfaces.

2. Locate the middle cerebellar peduncle (note its appearance on dorsal and ventral surfaces).

3. Note the relationship of the pons to the cerebellum.

4. Locate the area of the fourth ventricle on the brainstem specimen and the model with the cerebellum removed.

Midbrain

1. Note the rostral and caudal boundaries of the midbrain and the dorsal and ventral surfaces.

2. Locate:

    a. The cerebral peduncles and their outer covering, the crus cerebri

    b. The inferior and superior colliculi

    c. The interpeduncular fossa

    d. The superior cerebellar peduncles

Sagittal Sections: Cortex, Diencephalon, Brainstem

Using the sagittally sectioned specimens, review the structures that were identified on the whole brain and the brainstem. New structures that are visible will also be identified. It is important that you use both the whole brain and the sagittally sectioned brain together by finding the structure on each and comparing its appearance and location. This will help you achieve a three-dimensional concept of these structures.

In orienting yourself to the sagittal section, review the divisions of the brain, the lobes, the sulci, gyri, and fissures. The structures of the cortex, brainstem, and diencephalon will be reviewed below, and new structures will be added. Refer to Figure 2-3, *A* and *B*, to help visualize structures within each plane.

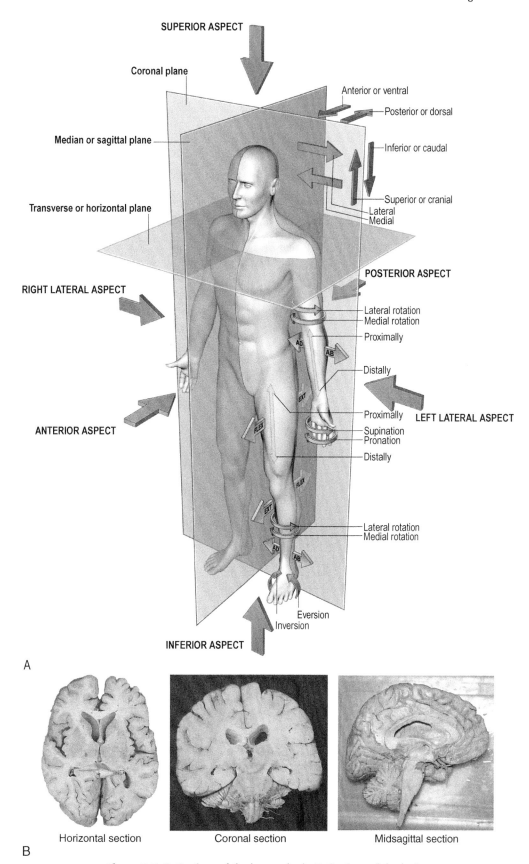

A

SUPERIOR ASPECT

Coronal plane

Median or sagittal plane

Transverse or horizontal plane

RIGHT LATERAL ASPECT

ANTERIOR ASPECT

Anterior or ventral
Posterior or dorsal
Inferior or caudal
Superior or cranial
Lateral
Medial
POSTERIOR ASPECT
Lateral rotation
Medial rotation
Proximally
Distally
Proximally   LEFT LATERAL ASPECT
Supination
Pronation
Distally
Lateral rotation
Medial rotation
Eversion
Inversion

INFERIOR ASPECT

B

Horizontal section   Coronal section   Midsagittal section

Figure 2-3 A, Sections of the human body. **B,** Sections of the brain.

Cortex

In sagittal section, review the following CNS structures and note their relationship to surrounding structures.

1. The corpus callosum

   a. What is the function of this structure?

   b. Note its relationship to the lateral ventricles.

   c. Locate the genu, body, splenium, and rostrum of the corpus callosum.

2. The cingulate gyrus

   a. Note the relationship of the cingulate gyrus to the corpus callosum.

   b. What would the corpus callosum, the lateral ventricles, and the cingulate gyrus look like if a mid-frontal or mid-coronal section were made through them on a whole brain?

3. Label the structures identified on Figure 2-4.

   A. _____

   B. _____

   C. _____

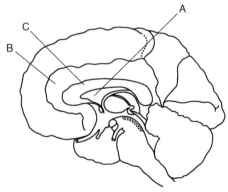

Figure 2-4 Midsagittal view of the brain.

4. The fornix

   a. Note the appearance of the fornix if it is visible on your specimen (or use a text to determine its location and relationship to the above structures).

   b. Note how the fornix begins as two parallel columns, which narrow as they travel anteriorly.

   c. What system does the fornix function in?

   d. In what structures does the fornix begin and end?

   e. What would the fornix look like if a frontal section was made at various places? (Hint: see Lundy-Ekman, p. 16, Figure 1-5.)

Diencephalon

1. Note the appearance of the diencephalon in sagittal section.

2. Locate the four divisions of the diencephalon and grossly note their boundaries.

   a. The thalamus

   b. The epithalamus (posterior to thalamus)

   c. The subthalamus (this is a deep structure and cannot be seen in saggital section)

    d. Hypothalamus (anterior to thalamus)

    e. The hypothalamic sulcus

        I. What parts of the diencephalon does this sulcus demarcate?

        II. What is the relationship of the third ventricle to the diencephalon?

3. Identify these structures in relation to the diencephalon.

    a. The mammillary body

    b. The infundibulum

    c. The optic chiasm

    d. The pineal gland

        I. What is the function and significance of this gland?

4. Visualize or make a drawing of the appearance of the third ventricle and the thalamus in a mid-frontal or mid-coronal section.

Cerebellum

1. Identify the vermis and the cortex of the cerebellum on the whole brain and in sagittal section.

2. Observe how each of the cerebellar peduncles connects with the cerebellum and review the function of each cerebellar peduncle (see Figure 2-5).

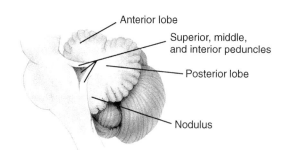

Anterior lobe

Superior, middle, and interior peduncles

Posterior lobe

Nodulus

Figure 2-5 Cerebellar peduncles.

Medulla

1. Note the appearance and boundaries of the medulla on the sagittal section.

2. What two midline landmarks of the medulla are cut to make the midsagittal section?

3. Note the relationship of the fourth ventricle and the central canal to the medulla.

4. Visualize or make a drawing of the ventricular system (central canal or fourth ventricle) at:

   a. The rostral medulla, near the pons-medulla junction

   b. The central canal

   c. The caudal medulla

5. Review the following medulla structures on the sagittal section. Identify whether the structures that are listed below are on the posterior or anterior aspect of the brainstem.

   a. The pyramids

   b. The fasciculus gracilis

   c. The fasciculus cuneatus

   d. The inferior olive

   e. The inferior cerebellar peduncle (if visible)

Pons

1. Note the appearance and boundaries of the pons in the sagittal section.

2. Note the relationship of the cerebellum to the pons.

3. What structure makes up the majority of the pons?

4. Note the relationship of the cerebral aqueduct and the fourth ventricle to the pons.

5. Visualize or make a drawing of the ventricular system (fourth ventricle) at:

   a. Low pons

   b. High pons

6. Identify the cerebellopontine angle.

Midbrain

1. Note the appearance of the midbrain in sagittal section and identify its ventral, dorsal, rostral, and caudal borders.

2. Identify:

   a. The cerebral peduncle (crus cerebri)

   b. The cerebral aqueduct

   c. The superior colliculi

   d. The inferior colliculi

3. Note that the cerebral aqueduct divides the midbrain into two divisions. What is the name of each division and what structures are contained in each?

4. Visualize the appearance of the cerebral aqueduct, the superior colliculi, and the cerebral peduncle in sagittal section. Make a rough sketch of your visualization and then check it against a picture in a text or refer to Figure 2-6 in this manual.

5. Label the structures identified on Figure 2-6.

A. _____

B. _____

C. _____

D. _____

E. _____

F. _____

G. _____

H. _____

I. _____

J. _____

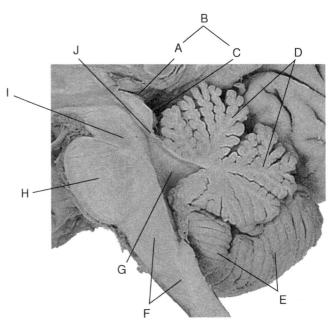

Figure 2-6 Sagittal section of the brainstem with cerebellum.

Cerebellum, Cranial Nerves, Ventricular System, and Spinal Cord Anatomy

Cerebellum, Cranial Nerves, Ventricular System, and Spinal Cord Anatomy

MATERIALS
Brain specimens, brain, ventricular and brainstem models, books, atlas

GOAL

The goal of this lab is to demonstrate an understanding of structures associated with the cerebellum, ventricular system, and spinal cord. Students will also be able to identify, locate, and define cranial nerves located on the brainstem.

PREPARATION FOR LAB

It takes 2 to 4 hours to prepare for this lab.
1. Complete the review of Lab 2. Most of the material will have been covered in the prior lab. Please reference your findings with page numbers. This will help you complete the lab in a timely fashion.
2. Use your textbooks and atlas as a reference. Indicate on each lab section the page number of the textbook showing photos of the structures in each section. Bring these texts to the lab to use as references. You may use the pictures in this lab manual to help you initially identify the structures on the specimen and in other texts.
3. Complete at least 25% of the picture labeling activity in the lab.
   Your lab instructor will check that you have prepared for the lab and will sign below.

_____

Signature of Lab Instructor

REVIEW OF LAB 2

1. Name the structure that is a band of fibers that transmits information between cerebral hemispheres.

2. The epithalamus consists of primarily what gland?

3. Which ventricle is located in the space between the thalami?

4. The tectum consists of what two structures?

5. List *five* structures located on the medulla.

6. The fasciculus gracilis carries _____ information.
7. The fasciculus cuneatus carries _____ information.

LAB 3

Cerebellum: Whole and Sagittal Views

The cerebellum (cb) is located dorsal to the brainstem. It consists of two cerebellar hemispheres and a midline vermis. It is helpful to use the sagittal sections with the whole brain to study the cerebellum sections. Note the relationship of the cerebellum to the brainstem, particularly the three cerebellar peduncles as they enter the cerebellum. Note the appearance and boundaries of the cerebellum, especially its relationship to the fourth ventricle.

1. Label the structures identified on Figure 3-1.

   A. _____

   B. _____

   C. _____

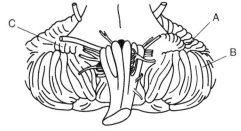

Figure 3-1 Gross anatomy of the cerebellum with brainstem (anterior view).

2. Label the structures identified on Figure 3-2.

A. _____

B. _____

C. _____

D. _____

E. _____

F. _____

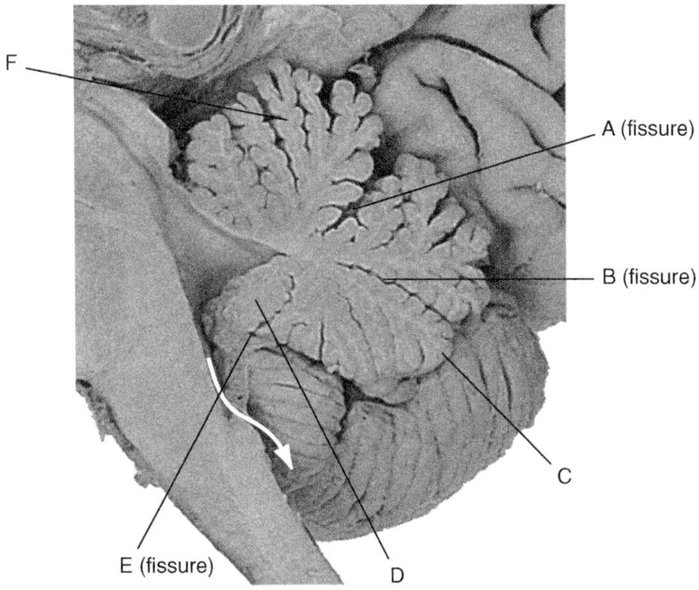

Figure 3-2 Gross anatomy of the cerebellum (sagittal view).

3. Label the structures identified on Figure 3-3.

A. _____

B. _____

C. _____

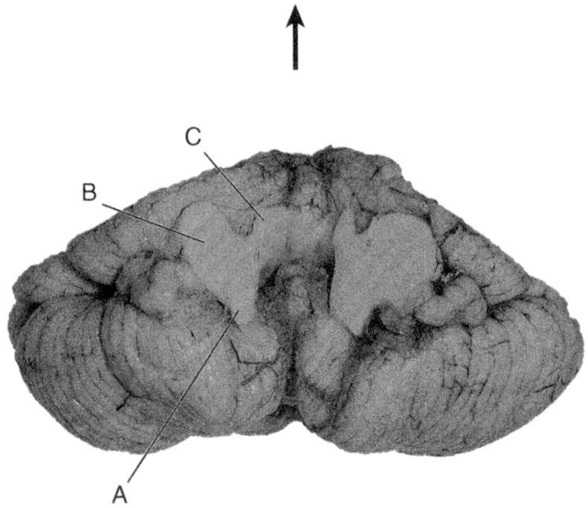

Figure 3-3 Ventral surface of the cerebellum (brainstem removed): cerebellar peduncles.

4. What is the general function of the cerebellum?

5. What is the function of the cerebellum?

7. On the external surface of the whole cerebellum on the sagittal section, locate the following:

    a. Lobes

        i. The anterior lobe—paleocerebellum

        ii. The posterior lobe—neocerebellum

        iii. The flocculonodular lobe

    b. Fissures

        i. The primary fissure

            1. What lobes does the primary fissure divide?

        ii. The horizontal fissure

        iii. The posterolateral fissure

            1. Which lobes does t.he posterolateral fissure divide?

    c. Other structures

        i. The vermis

            1. What structure does the vermis divide?

        ii. The cerebellar cortex

        iii. The inferior cerebellar peduncles

        iv. The middle cerebellar peduncles

        v. The superior cerebellar peduncles

8. Draw arrows on Figure 3-4 to indicate the direction of information traveling between the cerebellum and the brainstem.

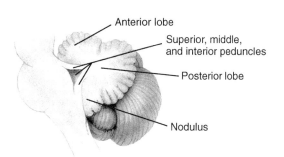

Figure 3-4 Cerebellar peduncles.

The lobes of the cerebellum are also named according to function. The **archicerebellum** is the phylogenetically oldest part of the cerebellum, and it evolved out of the vestibular system in organisms without limb buds; therefore, it is important in trunk control, and movement and equilibrium of the trunk.

The **anterior lobe**, or the **paleocerebellum**, developed in organisms with limb buds; therefore it is important in the control of extremity movement.

The newest part of the cerebellum is the **neocerebellum (posterior lobe)**, which developed in organisms with a cerebral cortex, so it is important in motor planning.

Cranial Nerves

1. Pneumonic Devices to help you learn the names and general function of each cranial nerve.

   Cranial Nerves: *O*h *O*h *O*h *T*o *T*ouch *A*nd *F*eel *V*ery *G*ood *V*egetables … *AH*!

   Sensory or Motor Function: *S*ome *S*ay *M*arry *M*oney *B*ut *M*y *B*rother *S*ays *B*ig *B*rains *M*atter *M*ore

2. Identify cranial nerves I through XII on a model, and then on the specimens.

3. Complete the table describing the cranial nerves.

Number	Name	Where the nerve exits the brainstem	Identify if the Nerve is Sensory or Motor and List Its Function
I.		Inferior frontal lobe	
II.		Diencephalon	
III.		Midbrain	
IV.		Posterior midbrain	
V.		Pons	
VI.		Pons/medulla	
VII.		Pons/medulla junction	
VIII.		Pons/medulla junction	
IX.		Medulla	
X.		Medulla	
XI.		Medulla	
XII.		Medulla	

4. Which cranial nerve originates on the dorsal surface of the brainstem?

5. Label the cranial nerves identified on Figure 3-5.

A. _____

B. _____

C. _____

D. _____

E. _____

F. _____

G. _____

H. _____

I. _____

J. _____

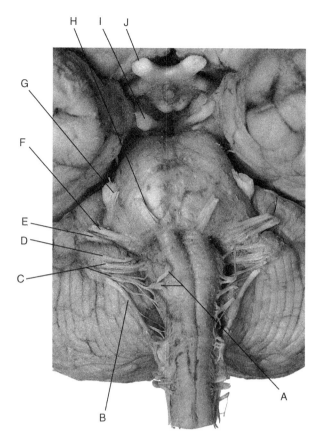

Figure 3-5 Anterior surface of the brainstem.

Ventricular System Model

MATERIALS
Ventricular model, sagittal view of the brain, and frontal or coronal sections.

The ventricular system consists of "spaces" in the brain and spinal cord, which contain cerebrospinal fluid. Use the model of the ventricular system to orient the location of the ventricular system within the brain and spinal cord.

It is necessary to understand the orientation of the ventricular system in the brain because it is used as a reference point in the study of the internal structures of the brain and brainstem.

1. Label the structures identified on Figure 3-6.

A. _____

B. _____

C. _____

D. _____

E. _____

F. _____

G. _____

H. _____

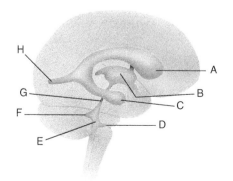

Figure 3-6 Lateral view of the ventricular system.

2. Label the structures identified on Figure 3-7.

A. _____

B. _____

C. _____

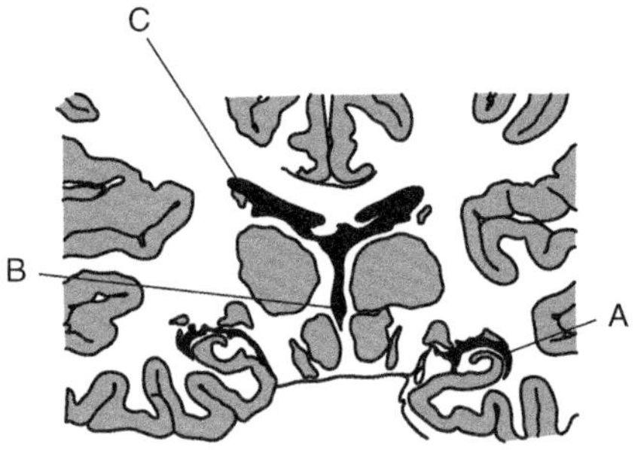

Figure 3-7 Coronal section displaying the ventricular system.

3. Use the model to locate the following structures. Identify the location (lobe and/or surrounding structures).

a. The two lateral ventricles

b. The anterior, central (body), inferior and posterior horns of the lateral ventricles

c. The interventricular foramen (of Monro)

d. The third ventricle

e. The cerebral aqueduct

f. The fourth ventricle

g. The two foramina of Luschka

h. The foramen of Magendie

The Ventricular System: Sagittal Section

On the sagittal section, locate the following parts of the ventricular system, and note their appearance and relationship to surrounding structures. Use the model of the ventricular system to orient yourself.

a. The lateral ventricles

b. Note the membrane that separates the two lateral ventricles: the septum pellucidum. Lift the septum and place your probe in the space lateral to it. What is this space?

c. Note the relationship of the corpus callosum to the lateral ventricles.

d. The third ventricle

    i. Locate the area where the third ventricle would be located. What structures surround and form the walls of the third ventricle?

e. The cerebral aqueduct

    i. Note how the aqueduct divides the midbrain into two divisions.

    ii. What are these divisions, and what structures are associated with each division?

    iii. In what shape would the aqueduct appear in a horizontal cross section?

f. The fourth ventricle

    i. What would the appearance of the fourth ventricle be if you made horizontal sections in various areas of the medulla and pons? Sketch your drawing below.

g. The two foramina of Luschka

h. The foramen of Magendie

    i. What is the function of the foramina of Luschka and Magendie?

i. The central canal

    i. What would the appearance of the central canal be if you made a horizontal section in the low medulla?

ii. What happens to the brain and skull when there is blockage or obstruction of the ventricular system in children? In adults?

iii. Where are the most common sites of blockage?

j. Locate the choroid plexus of the third, fourth, and lateral ventricles (may not be visible in all ventricles).

i. What is the function of the choroid plexus?

k. Try to visualize the appearance of the ventricular system as if a frontal (coronal) section was made through it in various places.

l. Explain how the CSF travels through the central nervous system.

5. Draw an arrow and label the structure of the ventricular system at the caudal medulla on Figure 3-8.

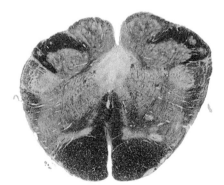

Figure 3-8 The caudal medulla.

6. Draw an arrow and label the structure of the ventricular system at the rostral medulla on Figure 3-9.

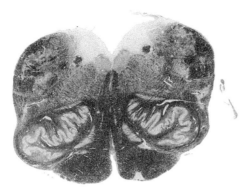

Figure 3-9 The rostral medulla.

7. Draw an arrow and label the structure of the ventricular system at the midpons on Figure 3-10.

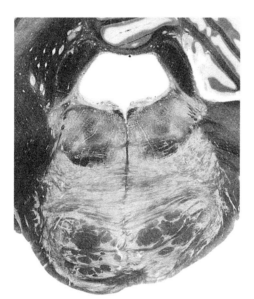

Figure 3-10 The midpons.

8. Draw an arrow and label the structure of the ventricular system at the caudal midbrain on Figure 3-11.

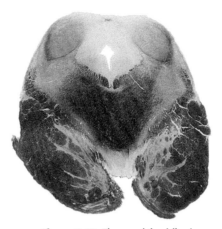

Figure 3-11 The caudal midbrain.

9. Draw an arrow and label the structure of the ventricular system at the rostral midbrain on Figure 3-12.

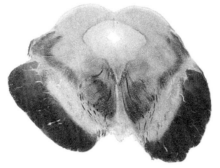

Figure 3-12 The rostral midbrain.

Spinal Cord Anatomy

MATERIALS
Spinal cord specimens, texts, model

Use Figure 3-13 while completing this lab. On the whole spinal cord specimens, identify the following:

1. Protective coverings of the spinal cord

    a. Dura mater

    b. Arachnoid mater

    c. Pia mater

2. Denticulate or dentate ligaments

3. Fissures and sulci of the spinal cord

    a. Anterior median fissure

    b. Dorsal median sulcus

    c. Dorsal intermediate sulcus

4. Roots and spinal nerves

    a. Dorsal rootlets

    b. Dorsal roots

    c. Ventral rootlets

    d. Ventral roots

    e. Spinal nerve

5. Distinct features of the spinal cord

    a. Conus medullaris

    b. Cauda equina

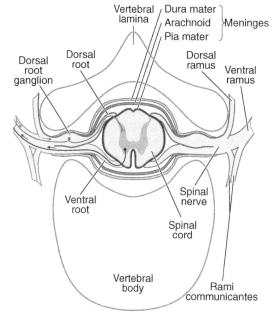

Figure 3-13 Spinal cord anatomy.

Spinal cord segments

The spinal cord is composed of 31 spinal cord segments (not vertebrae). There are 8 cervical, 12 thoracic, 5 lumbar, 5 sacral, and 1 coccygeal segment. Each group has distinguishing characteristics in cross-sectional view, such as size and shape of segment, amount of gray versus white matter, and the shape of the gray matter.

1. In the table below, describe the characteristics of each group of segments. Then draw a picture of each level to demonstrate its distinguishing characteristics.

	White vs. Gray Drawing	Shape (largest/smallest)	Sketch of Spinal Cord Segment
Distinguishing Characteristics/ Size (round, oval, etc.)			
Cervical			
Thoracic			
Lumbar			
Sacral			

2. The spinal cord ends at L1/L2 in the adult and the cauda equina begins. Draw a picture to note the relationship of the vertebral column to the spinal cord.

Cerebral and Diencephalic Internal Structures

Cerebral and Diencephalic Internal Structures

GOAL

MATERIALS
Brain specimens; whole, coronal, sagittal, and ventricular system models

The goal of this lab is to identify and locate internal structures of the cerebrum and diencephalon.

PREPARATION FOR LAB

1. Complete the review of Lab 3. Most of the material has been covered in the prior Lab. Please reference your findings with page numbers. This will help you complete the lab in a timely fashion.
2. Use your textbooks and atlas as a reference. Indicate on each lab section the page numbers of the textbook showing photos of the structures in each section. Bring these texts to the lab to use as references. You may use the pictures in this lab manual to help you initially identify the structures on the specimen and in other texts.
3. Complete at least 25% of the picture labeling activity in the lab.

Your lab instructor will check that you have prepared for the lab and will sign below.

_____

Signature of Lab Instructor

REVIEW OF LAB 3

1. Identify the lobes of the cerebellum.

2. Complete the following chart:

Number	Name	Level of the Brainstem that the Nerve Exits	Function
III.	Oculomotor		
IV.			Moves eye medially and down
VI.	Abducens		
XI.			Elevates shoulders and turns head

3. What is the consequence of a blockage or obstruction in the ventricular system in adults?

4. Identify the number of spinal cord segments in each section:

Cervical Section:

Thoracic Section:

Lumbar Section:

Sacral Section:

LAB 4

Coronal Sections

Use the coronal sections to identify the internal structures listed below. It is very important to use the coronal sections in series to get a three-dimensional picture of the structures. It is also important to use the coronal sections with the sagittal section and the whole brain to appreciate the location and relationship of structures to one another.

Certain structures are useful in orienting the coronal sections in terms of location and other structures. The ventricular system and the corpus callosum are very useful in this respect. Examine the ventricular system and the corpus callosum in series in each coronal section using the questions listed below as a guide. Refer to the ventricular system model as necessary.

1. Identify the ventricles present in each coronal section. (Be specific; i.e., identify which horn of the lateral ventricles is visible.)

2. What is the appearance of the ventricle(s)? Is this a change from the previous section? If so, how?

3. What is the appearance of the corpus callosum, and what is its relationship to the ventricles in each section?

4. Identify the lobe(s) of the brain in each coronal section.

In the next part of the lab session, you will look at the internal structures of the brain, brainstem, and cerebellum. Many of these structures were not visible or only partially visible on whole and sagittal section specimens. To visualize the three-dimensionality of these structures, it is important to review their appearance on whole and/or sagittal specimens and compare them to the coronal or cross-sectional appearance. Also note the relationship of surrounding structures.

Arc Structures

These structures are ones that follow the C-shape of the cortex. Study them in series, using the coronal section specimens with a picture from a text as a reference. Note the relationship of these structures to the ventricular system and the corpus callosum and how their appearance changes as you proceed through the sections, from frontal to occipital lobes.

We will study 5 series of arc structures: the lateral ventricles, the corpus callosum, cingulate and parahippocampal gyri, the uncus and the caudate nucleus, and the hippocampus-fornix-mammillary bodies. At this point, simply identify the structures and become aware of their course through the cortex. Later, we will study each arc structure as part of a cortical system.

The Lateral Ventricles: Anterior, Inferior and Posterior Horns

1. Locate the anterior horns in the frontal and parietal lobes.

2. Note the changes in shape of the anterior horns as they pass through the frontal and parietal lobes.

3. Locate the inferior horns in the temporal lobes.

4. Locate the posterior horns in the occipital lobes.

5. Locate the following ventricular structures in a midcoronal section.

    a. Anterior horn of the lateral ventricle

    b. Inferior horn of the lateral ventricle

    c. The third ventricle

6. Identify the lateral fissure

The Corpus Callosum

1. The corpus callosum is a C-shaped structure in the brain. Sketch its shape in the whole brain.

2. Note the relationship of the corpus callosum to the lateral ventricles in the coronal section.

The Cingulate Gyrus-Parahippocampal Gyrus-Uncus

1. Locate the cingulate gyrus and the parahippocampal gyrus in series on the coronal sections.

2. Compare the location and appearance of the cingulate gyri and the parahippocampal gyri on the sagittal and coronal sections.

3. Identify the relationship of the uncus to the parahippocampal gyrus in the sagittal section.

4. Note the relationship of the cingulate gyri to the medial longitudinal fissure and the corpus callosum on the coronal sections.

The Caudate Nucleus: Head, Body, and Tail

1. Note the relationship of the caudate nucleus to the lateral ventricles. In certain coronal sections, both the head and tail of the caudate are present (although the tail is often difficult to locate). If you cannot find the section where they are both visible, make sure you get an appreciation of this arc structure by visualizing how it curves through the cerebrum, looking at other specimens and referring to references.

2. What is the relationship of the head of the caudate to the lateral ventricles?

The Hippocampus, Fornix, and Mammillary Bodies

1. Note the appearance of the fornix as it arcs from the hippocampus to the mammillary bodies. Note how it changes from two separate columns to two adjoined columns to two separate columns again.

2. What is the relationship of the fornix to the lateral ventricles in terms of location?

3. The fornix is associated with which system?

4. What is the relationship of the hippocampus to the parahippocampal gyrus?

5. The hippocampus has the appearance of a seahorse when viewed from above, and thus the name hippocampus. What is the function of the hippocampus?

Other Internal Structures of the Cortex

Locate the following structures and note their relationship to the ventricular system and other nearby structures.

The Thalamus

1. Note its appearance in the coronal sections

2. Which ventricle is it located around? What is its orientation to this ventricle (medial, lateral, anterior, or posterior)?

The Basal Nuclei/Basal Ganglia

The basal ganglia are a group of subcortical nuclei that function in stereotyped movements and posture. Use a text and the coronal sections to locate these nuclei and the structures located near them. These nuclei are best seen on the coronal section where the third ventricle is present.

1. Locate them on the specimen.

    a. The globus pallidus

    b. The putamen

    c. The caudate nucleus

2. Define the following divisions of the basal ganglia in terms of what structures they contain.

    a. Striatum

    b. The lenticular (or lentiform) nuclei

3. Locate the following structures, which are listed from medial to latereal in a coronal section. Use a section where both lateral ventricles and the third ventricle are visible.

    a. The third ventricle

    b. The thalamus

    c. The internal capsule

    d. The globus pallidus

    e. The putamen

    f. The external capsule

    g. The claustrum

    h. The extreme capsule

    i. The insula

    j. The lateral fissure

4. Label the structures identified on Figure 4-1.

    A. _____

    B. _____

    C. _____

    D. _____

    E. _____

    F. _____

    G. _____

    H. _____

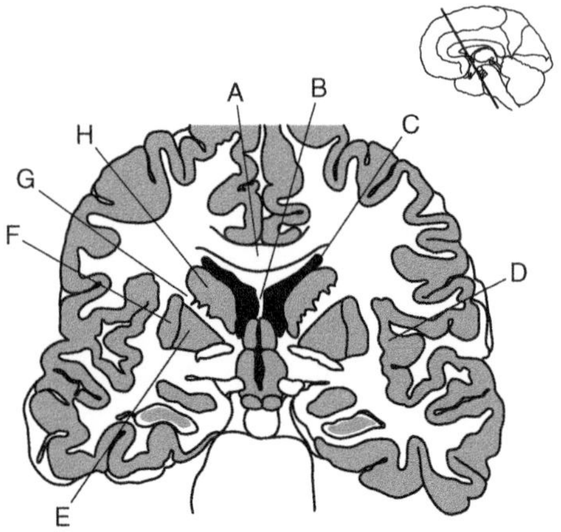

Figure 4-1 Coronal section through the frontal lobe.

5. Label the structures identified on Figure 4-2.

   A. _____

   B. _____

   C. _____

   D. _____

   E. _____

   F. _____

   G. _____

   H. _____

   I. _____

   J. _____

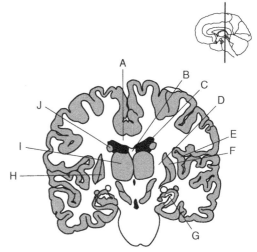

Figure 4-2 Coronal section.

6. Label the structures identified on Figure 4-3.

   A. _____

   B. _____

   C. _____

   D. _____

   E. _____

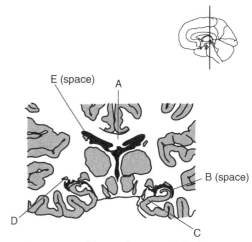

Figure 4-3 Midcoronal section of the brain.

Cerebellum: Horizontal Section View

1. Locate the deep nuclei of the cerebellum on Figure 4-4 below. It is not necessary to identify each nuclei separately..

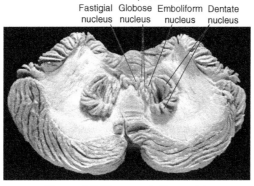

Figure 4-4 Deep cerebellar nuclei.

Brainstem Internal Structures

If necessary, briefly review the external structures of the brainstem on the models, using both the whole and sagittal brain.

Use pictures of the brainstem cross sections (found in Nolte, Haines and Lundy-Ekman) to locate the structures listed below and note their relationship to one another.

Note the appearance of the ventricular system in each cross section, as it is often used as a reference to identify the level of the cross section.

At the end of the lab, label the structures that you identified in the cross sections. (Note: There are also some cranial nerve nuclei that are visible on these sections. We will learn a few of them, which will assist you in our future study of cranial nerve nuclei.)

1. Low medulla (caudal medulla)

   a. What are the distinguishing features that cue you to identify this cross section? (i.e., shape, size, gray vs. white, etc.?)

   b. What is the appearance of the ventricular system?

   c. Draw the caudal medulla showing the appearance of the ventricular system

   d. Locate the:

       i. Anterior median fissure

       ii. The dorsal median sulcus

       iii. The dorsal intermediate sulcus

       iv. Pyramids

       v. Fasciculi gracilis and cuneatus

       vi. Nuclei gracilis and cuneatus

       vii. Medial lemniscus

       viii. Pyramidal decussation (if visible)

2. Rostral medulla (pons-medulla junction)

    a. What are the distinguishing features that orient you to the level of this section?

    b. What is the appearance of the ventricular system? Why?

    c. Draw the appearance of the ventricular system.

    d. Locate the:

        i. Anterior median fissure

        ii. The dorsal median sulcus

        iii. The dorsal intermediate sulcus

        iv. Pyramids

        v. Fasciculi gracilis and cuneatus

        vi. Nuclei gracilis and cuneatus

        vii. Medial lemniscus

        viii. Pyramidal decussation (if visible)

        ix. Inferior olivary nucleus

        x. Medial longitudinal fasciculus (MLF)

        xi. Hypoglossal nuclei of CN XII

3. Midpons

    a. What are the distinguishing features of this level?

    b. What is the appearance of the ventricular system?

c. Draw the appearance of the ventricular system.

d. Compare this with its appearance on the sagittal section.

e. Locate the:

     i. Middle cerebellar peduncle

     ii. Pontine nuclei

     iii. Medial lemniscus

     iv. Medial longitudinal fasciculus (MLF)

     v. Superior cerebellar peduncle

     vi. Abducens nuclei of CN VI (in the caudal pons)

4. The midbrain, inferior colliculi level (caudal)

a. What are the distinguishing features of this cross section?

b. Draw the appearance of the ventricular system.

c. Locate the:

     i. Inferior colliculi

     ii. Crus cerebri

     iii. Substantia nigra

     iv. Medial longitudinal fasciculus (MLF)

     v. Medial lemniscus

     vi. Trochlear nuclei of CN IV

5. The midbrain, superior colliculi level (rostral)

    a. What are the distinguishing features of this level?

    b. Draw the appearance of the ventricular system.

    c. Locate the:

       i. Crus cerebri

       ii. Substantia nigra

       iii. Red nucleus

       iv. Medial lemniscus

       v. MLF

       vi. Oculomotor nucleus of CN III

6. Draw lines and label the following structures of the caudal medulla on Figure 4-5.

    A. Anterior median fissure
    B. Dorsal median sulcus
    C. Dorsal intermediate sulcus
    D. Pyramids
    E. Fasciculus gracilis
    F. Fasciculus cuneatus
    G. Nucleus gracilis
    H. Nucleus cuneatus
    I. Medial lemniscus
    J. Central canal

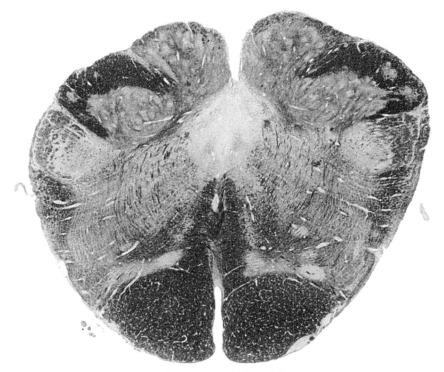

Figure 4-5 Caudal medulla.

7. Draw lines and label the following structures of the rostral medulla on Figure 4-6.

    A. Anterior median fissure
    B. Dorsal median sulcus
    C. Dorsal intermediate sulcus
    D. Pyramids
    E. Fasciculus gracilis
    F. Fasciculus cuneatus
    G. Nucleus gracilis
    H. Nucleus cuneatus
    I. Medial lemniscus
    J. Inferior olive
    K. Medial longitudinal fasciculus
    L. Fourth ventricle

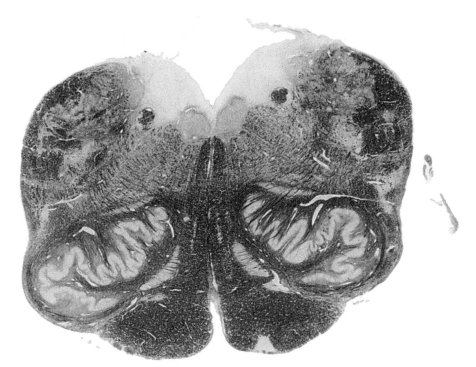

Figure 4-6 Rostral medulla.

8. Draw lines and label the following structures of the midpons on Figure 4-7.

    A. Medial longitudinal fasciculus
    B. Medial lemniscus
    C. Middle cerebellar peduncle
    D. Pontine nuclei
    E. Corticospinal and corticobulbar tracts
    F. Fourth ventricle

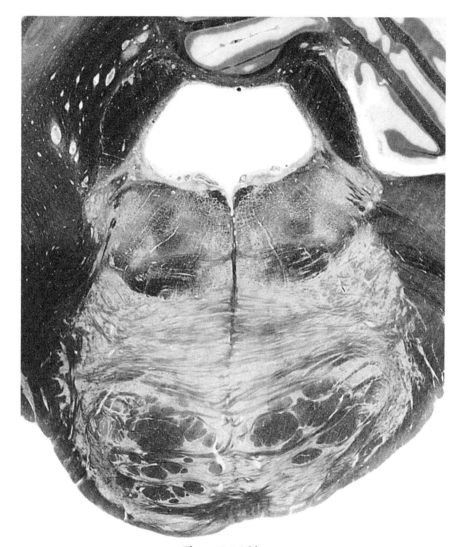

Figure 4-7 Midpons.

9. Draw lines and label the following structures of the caudal midbrain on Figure 4-8.

    A. Medial longitudinal fasciculus
    B. Medial lemniscus
    C. Crus cerebri
    D. Inferior colliculi
    E. Substantia nigra
    F. Trochlear nuclei of CN IV
    G. Cerebral aqueduct

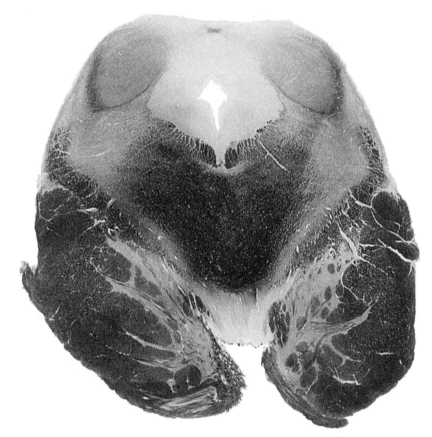

Figure 4-8 Caudal midbrain.

10. Draw lines and label the following structures of the rostral midbrain on Figure 4-9.

    A. Crus cerebri
    B. Red nucleus
    C. Substantia nigra
    D. Medial lemniscus
    E. Medial longitudinal fasciculus
    F. Oculomotor nuclei of CN III
    G. Superior colliculi
    H. Cerebral aqueduct

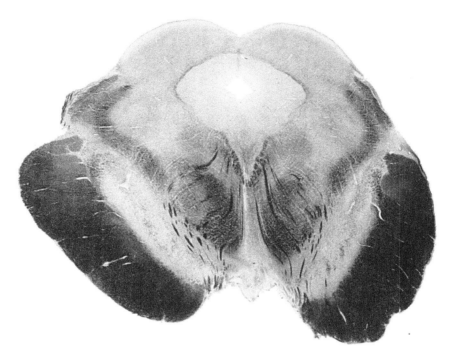

Figure 4-9 Rostral midbrain.

5

Meninges, Blood Vessels, and Cranium

Meninges, Blood Vessels, and Cranium

MATERIALS
Brain specimens, whole brain model, atlas, cranium

GOAL

The goal of this lab is for students to identify the major blood vessels that supply the brain and spinal cord, identify the three protective coverings, and identify the specific bones of the skull that serve to protect the brain.

PREPARATION FOR LAB

1. Complete the review of Lab 4. Most of the material has been covered in the prior lab. Please reference your findings with page numbers. This will help you complete the lab in a timely fashion.
2. Complete the case story before the lab.
3. Use your textbooks and atlas as a reference. Indicate on each lab section the page number of the textbook showing photos of the structures in each section. Bring these texts to the lab to use as references. You may use the pictures in this lab manual to help you initially identify the structures on the specimen and in other texts.
4. Complete at least 25% of the picture labeling activity in the lab.

Your lab instructor will check that you have prepared for the lab and will sign below.

_____

Signature of Lab Instructor

REVIEW OF LAB 4

1. What is the function of the hippocampus?

2. Where is the uncus located?

3. What is the function of the globus pallidus and putamen?

4. Name three deep nuclei of the cerebellum.

5. What structure separates the fasciculus gracilis and fasciculus cuneatus?

6. Name the structure of the ventricular system that is located posterior to the pons?

7. The crus cerebri is the outer covering of what structure?

LAB 5

CASE STORY

Nancy is a 27-year-old female who was in a serious car accident. The car she was driving was hit on the passenger side, causing Nancy's head to thrust against the driver's side window. This resulted in a traumatic head injury. Using your knowledge of neuroanatomy, answer the following questions related to Nancy and traumatic head injury:

1. What area of the skull is most likely to be fractured due to this type of trauma, and why?

2. What protective structures does the brain have to decrease the forces of subsequent damage to the brain in an injury such as this?

3. Explain how the brain sits in the skull and how this may be disrupted during an impact such as Nancy's?

4. If an epidural hematoma results, explain where this may occur, how it may occur, what damage may occur to the brain, and what the symptoms of such a complication may be?

Protective Coverings of the Brain and Spinal Cord

In this lab, study the structures that protect and cover the brain. These include the meninges and skull.

The Meninges

There are three meninges that cover the brain: the dura mater, the arachnoid, and the pia mater.

Dura Mater

1. The dura mater has most likely been removed from the specimens. If there is a specimen available, note the thickness and appearance of this meninges. To what does the dura mater adhere?

2. There are two potential spaces associated with the dura: one above the dura and one below it.

   a. What are the names of these spaces?

   b. What is the clinical significance of these spaces in relation to a head or brain injury?

3. Note the differences between the epidural and subdural hematomas

	Blood Supply Involved	**Progression of Symptoms**
Epidural hematoma		
Subdural hematoma		

4. There are two main projections of dura: the falx cerebri and the tentorium cerebelli. Note the usual location of these on the brain (they may be visible in some specimens). What is the function of these?

Arachnoid

1. Note the arachnoid is attached to the surface of the whole brain. Lift a portion of it with a blunt instrument and note the weblike projections that attach the arachnoid to the brain. Note the subarachnoid space below the arachnoid. What is contained in this space? (This space collapses when the brain is removed.)

2. What is the major function of the arachnoid?

3. In some areas, the subarachnoid space is larger, and these areas are called cisterns. Of particular importance is the cisterna magnum (also referred to as the cerebellomedullary cistern), which is often used to receive excess CSF from an implanted shunt. Locate the area of the cisterna magnum on a sagittal specimen.

Pia Mater

1. The pia mater is adherent to the CNS and follows the contours of it. You are unable to lift it as you did the arachnoid mater. Observe the pia on the surface of the brain and note how it dips into the sulci and fissures.

Cranium and Cranial Cavity

1. Using the skulls, locate the following:

   a. Coronal suture

   b. Sagittal suture

   c. Temporal suture

   d. Occipital suture

2. Bones and landmarks of the skull

   a. Frontal bone

   b. Parietal bone

   c. Occipital bone

   d. Temporal bone

   e. Sphenoid bone

   f. Zygomatic bone (arch and process)

   g. Maxilla

   h. Mandible

   i. External acoustic meatus

   j. Mastoid process

   k. Occipital protuberance

3. Fossas

   a. What lobe and/or structures are cradled or found in each fossa?

      i. Anterior

      ii. Middle

      iii. Posterior

      iv. Foramen magnum

   b. How does the dura mater assist the skull in the protection of the cerebrum and cerebellum?

4. Label the structures identified on Figure 5-1.

A. _____

B. _____

C. _____

D. _____

E. _____

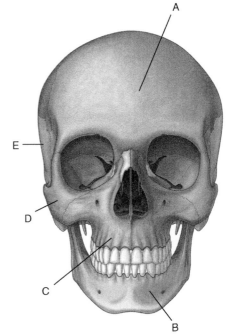

Figure 5-1 Anterior aspect of the skull.

5. Label the structures identified on Figure 5-2.

A. _____

B. _____

C. _____

D. _____

E. _____

F. _____

G. _____

H. _____

I. _____

J. _____

K. _____

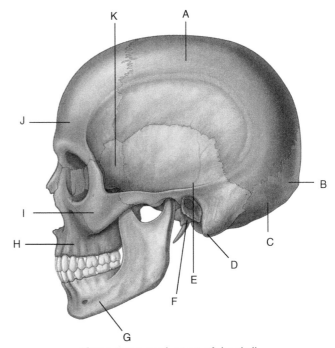

Figure 5-2 Lateral aspect of the skull.

6. Label the structures identified on Figure 5-3.

A. _____

B. _____

C. _____

D. _____

E. _____

F. _____

G. _____

H. _____

I. _____

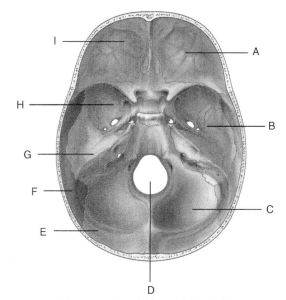

Figure 5-3 Cranial base of the skull.

Blood Vessels of the Brain

1. Examine the inferior surface of the whole brain. Identify:

   a. Vertebral arteries

   b. Anterior spinal artery

   c. Basilar artery

   d. Pontine (circumferential) arteries

   e. Superior cerebellar arteries

   f. Internal carotid arteries

   g. Posterior cerebral arteries

   h. Posterior communicating arteries

   i. Anterior communicating artery

   j. Anterior cerebral arteries

   k. Middle cerebral arteries

   l. Posterior inferior cerebellar arteries

   m. Anterior inferior cerebellar arteries

   n. Posterior spinal arteries

2. Identify those arteries that are part of the circle of Willis. What is the function of the circle of Willis?

3. Label the structures identified on Figure 5-4.

A. _____

B. _____

C. _____

D. _____

E. _____

F. _____

G. _____

H. _____

I. _____

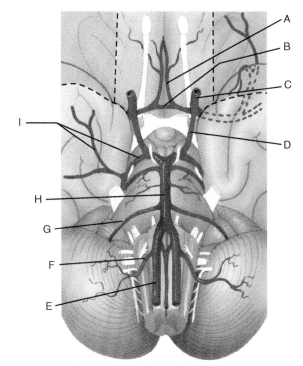

Figure 5-4 Blood vessels of the brain.

Midcoronal Section

1. Note which areas are supplied by the anterior, middle, and posterior cerebral arteries and what areas of the sensory and motor homunculus are located in these areas.

2. Identify the sensory and/or motor signs that result from an occlusion or hemorrhage to the following arteries.

	Sensory Signs	**Motor Signs**
Anterior cerebral artery		
Middle cerebral artery		
Posterior cerebral artery		

3. Locate the middle cerebral artery on a midcoronal section. Use your atlas first, then find it on specimens in the lab.

4. Label what artery would be found in the identified space on Figure 5-5.

A. _____

B. _____

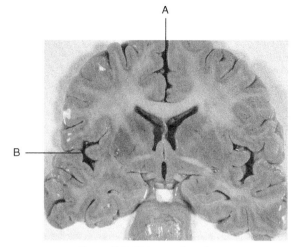

Figure 5-5 Midcoronal section.

5. Refer to the picture of the lateral, sagittal, and inferior views of the cerebrum (Figure 5-6). Color and label the blood supply to the major areas for the following anterior cerebral artery, middle cerebral artery, and posterior cerebral artery. Note: You may want to use a different color to shade in each artery's distribution. Figure 5-6.

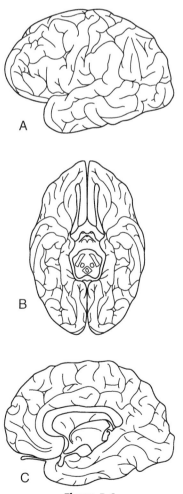

Figure 5-6

Muscle Spindle, GTO, and other Proprioceptors

Muscle Spindle, GTO, and other Proprioceptors

GOAL

The goal for this lab is for students to (1) identify the structures and functions associated with golgi tendon organs (GTO) and muscle spindle, as well as their contributions to normal and abnormal muscle tone, posture, and movement; and (2) to outline the basic circuitry for specific spinal cord reflexes associated with these functions. After a review of the anatomy and neurophysiology of the muscle spindle, GTO, and other spinal reflexes, students will apply this knowledge by answering questions from case stories to understand how the muscle spindle, GTO, and other spinal cord reflexes contribute to posture and movement, and how neurological symptoms are associated with spinal cord reflexes.

Your lab instructor will check that you have prepared for the lab and will sign below.

Signature of Lab Instructor

DRAW THE MUSCLE SPINDLE, GOLGI TENDON ORGAN, AND GAMMA MOTOR NEURON CIRCUITRY

On the following pages, complete the following activities:

- Activity 1: Draw and label the neuromuscular components that comprise the muscle spindle complex: include the nuclear bag, nuclear chain, IA endings, II endings, GTO and its synapse with the extrafusal muscle fiber, alpha motor neuron, gamma motor neuron and its synapse with the intrafusal muscle fiber, and pertinent interneurons involved in the aforementioned spinal reflexes.
- Activity 2: Draw and explain the circuitry of the phasic stretch (monosynaptic) reflex.
- Activity 3: Draw and explain the circuitry of the GTO.
- Activity 4: Draw and explain the circuitry of reciprocal inhibition.
- Activity 5: Draw and explain alpha and gamma co-activation. Explain its functional significance.

You may also wish to draw and explain how proprioceptive information from the muscle spindle and GTO travels to the cerebellum.

Activity 1: Muscle Spindle Complex

Draw and label the neuromuscular components that comprise the muscle spindle complex on Figure 6-1. Include the:

- Nuclear bag
- Nuclear chain
- Ia endings
- II endings
- GTO and its synapse with the extrafusal muscle fiber
- Alpha motor neuron
- Gamma motor neuron and its synapse with the intrafusal muscle fiber
- Pertinent interneurons involved in the aforementioned spinal reflexes

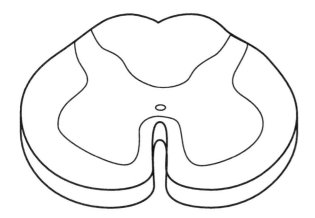

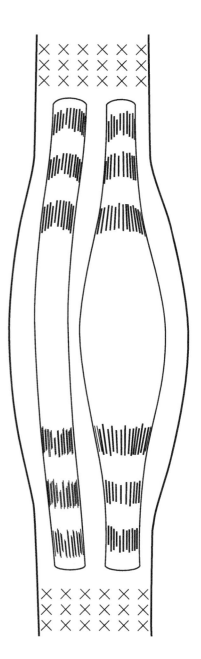

Figure 6-1

Activity 2: Phasic Stretch (Monosynaptic) Reflex

1. Draw and explain the circuitry of the phasic stretch (monosynaptic) reflex[1] on Figure 6-2.

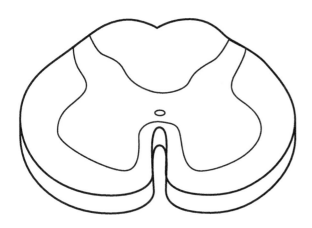

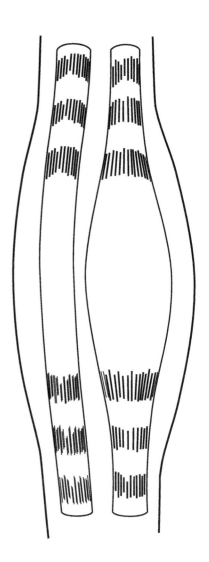

Figure 6-2

[1]Historically, the phasic stretch reflex was thought to play a significant role in spasticity; however, this view has changed in recent years. Refer to Lundy-Ekman Chapter 9, Motor System, for more details.

Activity 3: GTO Circuitry

1. Draw and explain the circuitry of the GTO on Figure 6-3.

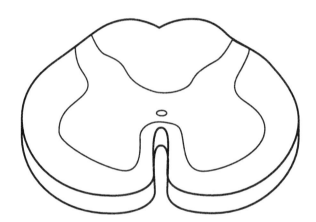

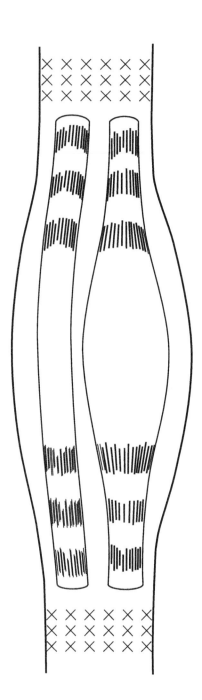

Figure 6-3

Activity 4: Reciprocal Inhibition

1. Draw and explain the circuitry of reciprocal inhibition on Figure 6-4.

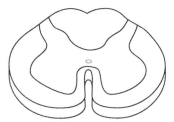

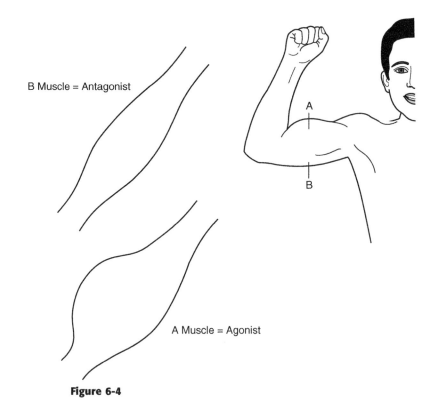

B Muscle = Antagonist

A Muscle = Agonist

Figure 6-4

Activity 5: Alpha-Gamma Co-Activation

1. Draw and explain alpha and gamma co-activation. Explain its functional significance.

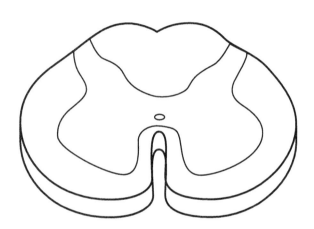

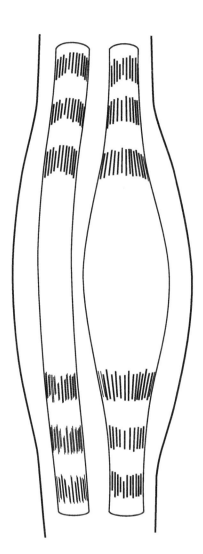

Figure 6-5

LAB QUESTIONS and CASE STORIES

Work in your small groups to answer the following questions.

1. How do the muscle spindle, GTO, and joint afferent contribute to normal movement and posture?

2. a. Refer to Figure 6-2 the phasic stretch reflex and describe how it functions.

   b. How is testing for the phasic stretch reflex done during a physical examination?

   c. How are phasic stretch reflexes used diagnostically?

d. Describe what is meant by the term *increased deep tendon reflexes*, including clinical implications.

3. What are the secondary endings of the muscle spindle and what conditions facilitate them? What are the neural components of the tonic stretch reflex and how does it function? Under what conditions can the tonic stretch reflex be elicited? Describe the circuitry of the tonic stretch reflex after an upper motor neuron (UMN) lesion?

4. The gamma motoneurons are the motor innervation to the muscle spindle receptors.

   a. Where are the cell bodies for the gamma motoneuron and what part of the muscle spindle does the gamma motor neuron innervate?

   b. Outline the circuitry.

    c. What causes the gamma motor neuron to activate?

5. What role does reciprocal inhibition play during normal movement? Explain the phenomenon of reciprocal inhibition, its circuitry, and its function in the nervous system.

6. A therapist is working with a patient who presents with spasticity in an extremity, resulting from a spinal cord injury. What role does reciprocal inhibition play when the therapist facilitates activity in the non-spastic muscle during feeding activity?

7. Explain the role of the GTO in functional activity during normal movement. Outline its circuitry.

8. What is muscle tone? What is the difference between hypotonia and hypertonia?

9. Identify the neural and myoplastic factors that contribute to muscle hyperstiffness during active movements in the following clinical populations: post-stroke, chronic spinal cord injury, and spastic cerebral palsy.

10. Melvin sustained a stroke two years ago. As a result, he presents with increased muscle stiffness in the left upper and lower extremities. At the age of 84, he continues to live with his wife in an apartment within an assistive living facility. He requires supervision with his activities of daily living; he ambulates with a hemiwalker at home and in the community. He enjoys reading books, going to the movies with his wife, and playing with his grandchildren. Each day, Melvin attends "morning exercises," where he receives personal attention from the therapy staff. Each day, the therapist performs passive range of motion on his left arm and leg.

    Explain the rationale for a therapist to perform *passive* range of motion on a client who had a stroke several years ago, demonstrates muscle stiffness in the affected extremity, and leads an active lifestyle.

11. Heather is a 31-year-old woman who sustained a traumatic brain injury as a result of a motor vehicle accident. Although she was awake when the paramedics came, she was unconscious by the time she arrived at the hospital. She was rushed to the intensive care unit (ICU), where she was medically stabilized. After 3 days in the ICU, the doctor ordered an OT/PT therapy evaluation. The therapy team evaluated Heather and determined that she required daily skilled services. A common therapeutic intervention for a client who is unconscious and dependent on a ventilator includes passive range of motion.

    Explain the rationale for a therapist to perform passive range of motion on this particular client, who is unconscious.

12. A patient with cerebrovascular accident (CVA) has extensor stiffness in his lower extremity, which causes his foot to go into plantar flexion. A common therapeutic technique is to place a splint known as a molded ankle-foot orthosis (MAFO) on the affected leg, which holds the foot in neutral. First, explain the mechanisms that might result in muscle shortening if the ankle is allowed to remain in the plantar flexed position. Second, using neurophysiological rationale, explain why this strategy may reduce muscle resistance. Third, explain the mechanisms that may be contributing to the patient's extensor muscle stiffness.

13. When a person presents with an upper extremity flexor spasticity synergy (elbow and wrist flexion with digits flexed and shoulder abducted), a common technique is to place a resting hand splint into their affected hand to reduce spasticity and elongate the muscle. Using neurophysiological rationale, explain why this may be an effective technique.

14. Gladyse sustained a CVA (right precentral gyrus/frontal lobe) a few months ago, resulting in flexor spasticity of her left upper extremity and extensor spasticity of her left lower extremity. She uses a wheelchair for mobility in her home and within the community. Although her wheelchair has a footrest, her foot frequently dangles. The foot spontaneously begins to "bounce" up and down uncontrollably. This is called clonus. Explain the neurophysiological rationale circuitry for this phenomenon.

15. What is the clasp-knife phenomenon? What neural mechanisms might be contributing to this experience? In what populations might you observe this sign?

Sensory Pathways

Sensory Pathways

GOAL

The goal of this lab is to identify the structures involved in each sensory pathway, trace each pathway, and state the function of each major sensory pathway. Lastly, students will identify symptoms associated with a unilateral lesion of each sensory pathway at the levels of the spinal cord, brainstem, and cerebral cortex.

PREPARATION FOR LAB

1. Prior to arriving at lab, prepare the drawings of the *sensory* pathways listed below using the worksheets provided (see following pages for details).

2. Indicate the page number of a text that shows the pathways indicated below. Place the page number next to the pathway below.

3. Bring these texts and pathway drawings to lab.

4. Sensory pathways are noted on the following pages and below:

   Conscious Sensory Pathways

   Dorsal column-medial lemniscal

   Lateral Spinothalamic

   Trigeminothalamic pathways (discriminative touch and conscious proprioception)

   Unconscious Sensory Pathways

   Anterior spinocerebellar

   Posterior spinocerebellar

   Rostral Spinocerebellar

   Cuneocerebellar

5. In class: After drawing and reviewing each sensory pathway, begin the Sensory Pathways and Case Stories Worksheet located at the end of Lab 7.

Your lab instructor will check that you have prepared for the lab and will sign below.

_____

Signature of Lab Instructor

LAB 7: PATHWAY DRAWING ASSIGNMENT

A. For each of the pathways listed (trigeminothalamic tract, dorsal column-medial lemniscal, lateral spinothalamic):
   1. Draw the pathway from receptor to cortex
   2. State the function of the pathway
   3. State (and show in drawing) where it crosses
   4. Indicate the symptoms that will manifest with a unilateral lesion in the:
      a. Spinal cord
      b. Brainstem
      c. Cortex
B. For each of the pathways listed (anterior spinocerebellar, cuneocerebellar, posterior spinocerebellar, rostral spinocerebellar):
   1. Draw the pathway from receptor to cortex
   2. State the function of the pathway
   3. State (and show in the drawing) where it crosses

Dorsal Column-Medial Lemniscal Pathway

1. Draw the pathway from receptor to cortex on Figure 7-1.

2. State the function.

3. State where the pathway crosses.

4. State the symptoms that will manifest with a unilateral lesion in the:

    a. Spinal cord

    b. Brainstem

    c. Cortex

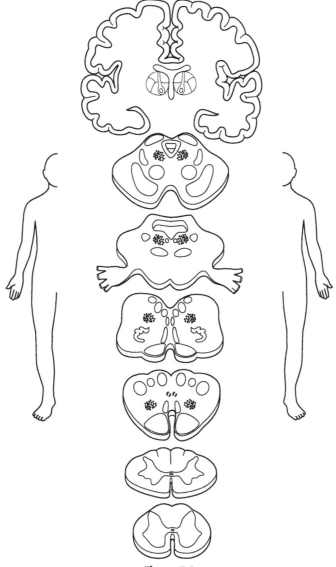

Figure 7-1

Spinothalamic Pathway

1. Draw the pathway from receptor to cortex on Figure 7-2.

2. State the function.

3. State where the pathway crosses.

4. State the symptoms that will manifest with a unilateral lesion in the:

   a. Spinal cord

   b. Brainstem

   c. Cortex

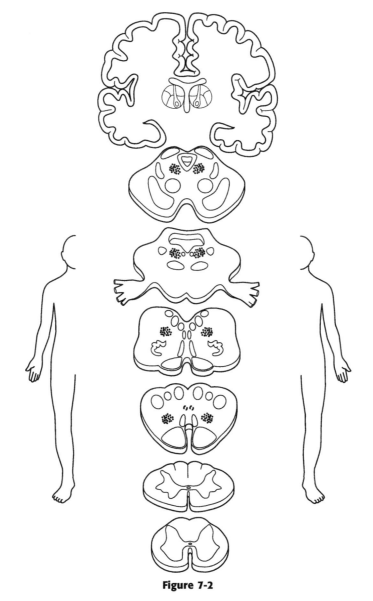

Figure 7-2

Trigeminothalamic Tract (Discriminative Touch and Conscious Proprioception) Pathway

1. Draw the pathway from receptor to cortex on Figure 7-3.

2. State the function.

3. State where the pathway crosses.

4. State the symptoms that will manifest with a unilateral lesion in the:

   a. Spinal cord

   b. Brainstem

   c. Cortex

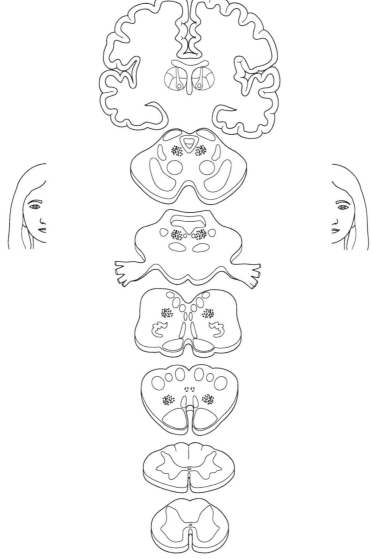

Figure 7-3

Anterior Spinocerebellar Pathway

1. Draw the pathway from receptor to cortex on Figure 7-4.

2. State the function.

3. State where the pathway crosses.

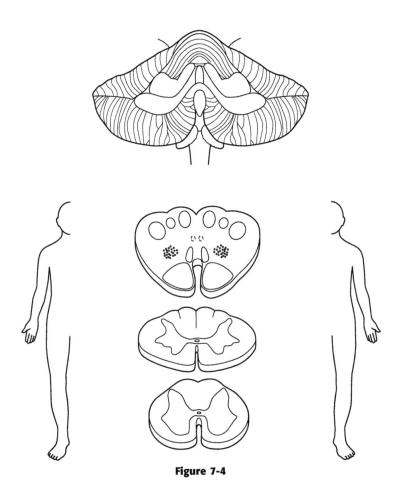

Figure 7-4

Cuneocerebellar Pathway

1. Draw the pathway from receptor to cortex on Figure 7-5.

2. State the function.

3. State where the pathway crosses.

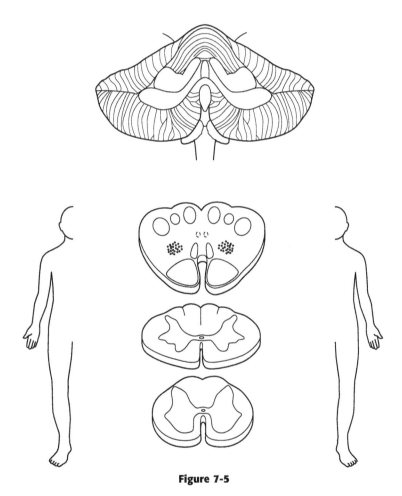

Figure 7-5

Posterior Spinocerebellar Pathway

1. Draw the pathway from receptor to cortex on Figure 7-6

2. State the function.

3. State where the pathway crosses.

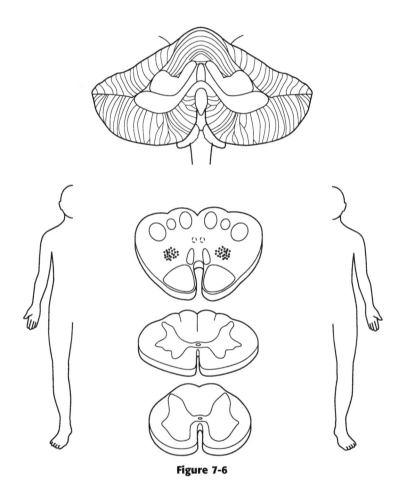

Figure 7-6

Rostral Spinocerebellar Pathway

1. Draw the pathway from receptor to cortex on Figure 7-7.

2. State the function.

3. State where the pathway crosses.

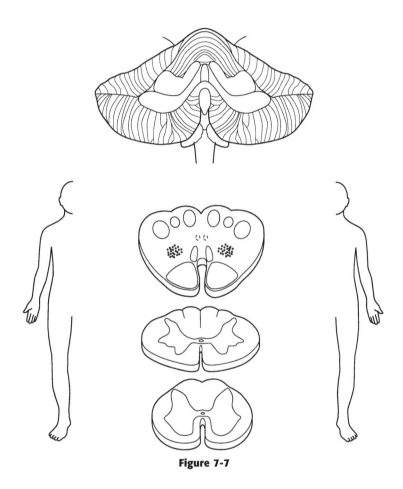

Figure 7-7

Sensory Pathways And Case Stories Worksheet

Please answer the following questions once you have completed your sensory pathways.

1. Identify the sensory pathway that relays information pertaining to pain and temperature.

2. Identify the pathway that travels in the medial lemniscus through the brainstem.

3. Why are there several pathways carrying proprioceptive information to the cerebellum?

4. Please read the case story and complete the table below. You may find it helpful to sketch a drawing of a spinal cord cross section and indicate the area of the lesion:

Mary is an 8-year-old girl who sustained a spinal cord injury at the level of C5. It is a complete lesion. What sensory deficits would you expect to find?

Sensory Pathway			Identify as Either Intact or Loss (and describe)	Summary of Symptoms Based Upon the Location of the Lesion: Bilateral, Ipsilateral, Contralateral
DCML	At the level of C5	Right side		
		Left side		
	Below the level of the lesion	Right side		
		Left side		
Spinothalamic	At the level of C5	Right side		
		Left side		
	Below the level of the lesion	Right side		
		Left side		

5. Please read the case story and complete the following table:

Peter is a 21-year-old man who accidentally fell off a ladder and sustained an incomplete spinal cord injury. A CAT scan revealed a lesion on the right side of the T8 spinal cord segment. What sensory symptoms would you expect?

Sensory Pathway			Identify as Either Intact or Loss (and describe)	Summary of Symptoms Based Upon the Location of the Lesion: Bilateral, Ipsilateral, Contralateral
DCML	At the level of T8	Right side		
		Left side		
	Below the level of the lesion	Right side		
		Left side		
Spinothalamic	At the level of T8	Right side		
		Left side		
	Below the level of the lesion	Right side		
		Left side		

6. Using the above case story, will Peter demonstrate any sensory deficits in his upper trunk and upper extremities?

7. Which sensory pathway carries discriminative touch from the face to the brain?

8. The third order neuron for both the DCML and the spinothalamic begins in the _____ and travels through the _____ and ends in the _____.

9. The spinocerebellar pathways carry _____ information that is processed in the _____.

10. True or False: The receptors for the spinocerebellar pathways include the muscle spindle and the Golgi tendon organ.

Motor Pathways

Motor Pathways

GOAL

The goal of this lab is to identify the structures that make up each motor pathway and state the function of each major motor pathway. Students will be able to identify symptoms associated with a unilateral lesion at the levels of the spinal cord, brainstem, and cerebral cortex.

PREPARATION FOR LAB

1. Prior to lab, prepare the drawings of the *motor* pathways on the worksheets provided (see following pages for details).

   Lateral Activating Pathways

   Lateral corticospinal

   Lateral reticulospinal

   Rubrospinal

   Corticobulbar

   Medial Activating Pathways

   Medial corticospinal

   Tectospinal

   Medial/anterior vestibulospinal

   Medial reticulospinal

   Lateral vestibulospinal

2. Indicate the page number of a text that shows the pathways indicated below. Place the page number next to the pathways.

3. Bring texts and pathway drawings to class.

4. Lab activity: After your drawings are finished, complete the Lab 8 Worksheet to review the information.

Your lab instructor will check that you have prepared for the lab and will sign below.

_____

Signature of Lab Instructor

PATHWAY ASSIGNMENT (Part I of II)

Complete and bring drawings to class to be reviewed.

For each of the following pathways (lateral corticospinal, medial corticospinal, corticobulbar):

a. Draw the pathway from the cortex to the body.

b. State the function of the pathway.

c. State (and show in drawing) where it crosses.

d. What symptoms will manifest with a unilateral lesion in:
   I. Spinal cord
   II. Brainstem
   III. Cortex

Lateral Corticospinal Pathway

1. Draw the pathway from cortex to body on Figure 8-1.

2. State the function.

3. State where the pathway crosses.

4. State the symptoms that will manifest with a unilateral lesion in the:

   a. Spinal cord

   b. Brainstem

   c. Cortex

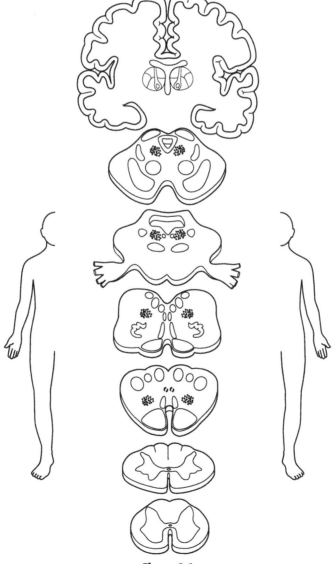

Figure 8-1

Medial Corticospinal Pathway

1. Draw the pathway from cortex to body on Figure 8-2.

2. State the function.

3. State where the pathway crosses.

4. State the symptoms that will manifest with a unilateral lesion in the:

    a. Spinal cord

    b. Brainstem

    c. Cortex

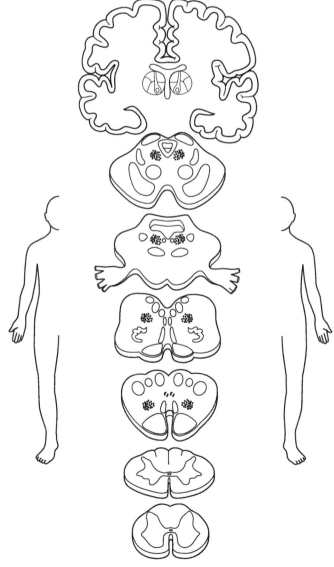

Figure 8-2

Corticobulbar Pathway

1. Draw the pathway from cortex to head on Figure 8-3.

2. State the function.

3. State where the pathway crosses.

4. State the symptoms that will manifest with a unilateral lesion.

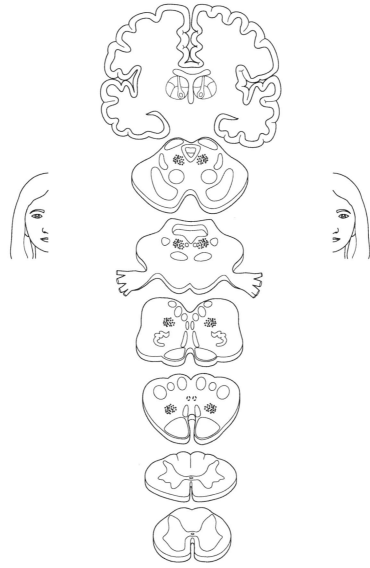

Figure 8-3

PATHWAY ASSIGNMENT (Part II of II)

Complete and bring drawings to class to be reviewed.

For each of the following pathways (lateral reticulospinal, rubrospinal, tectospinal, medial/anterior vestibular, lateral vestibular):

    a. Draw the pathway from cortex to body.
    b. State the function of the pathway.
    c. State (and show in drawing) where it crosses.

Tectospinal Pathway

1. Draw the pathway from cortex to body on Figure 8-4.

2. State the function.

3. State where the pathway crosses.

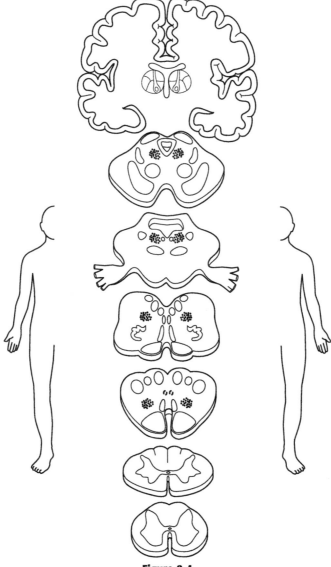

Figure 8-4

Lateral Vestibulospinal Pathway

1. Draw the pathway on Figure 8-5.

2. State the function.

3. State where the pathway crosses.

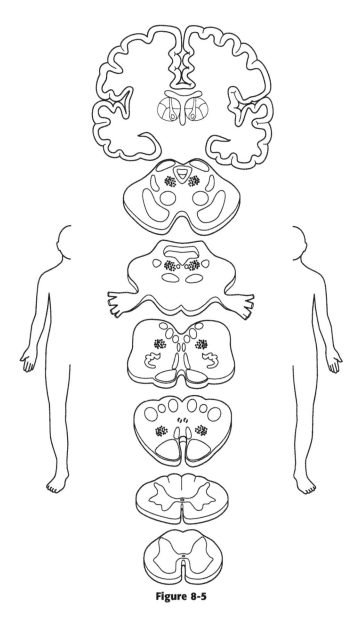

Figure 8-5

Medial Vestibulospinal Pathway

1. Draw the pathway from cortex to body on Figure 8-6:

2. State the function.

3. State where the pathway crosses.

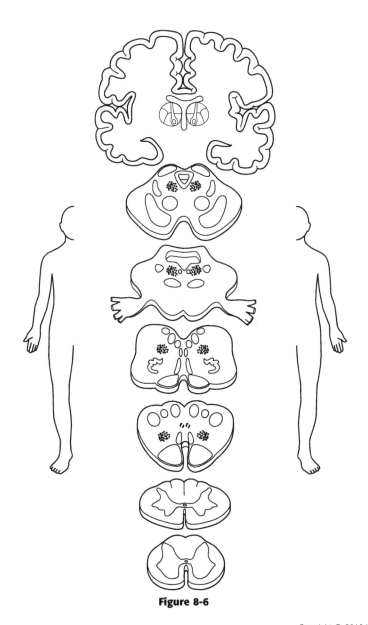

Figure 8-6

Medial Reticulospinal Pathway

1. Draw the pathway from cortex to body on Figure 8-7.

2. State the function.

3. State where the pathway crosses.

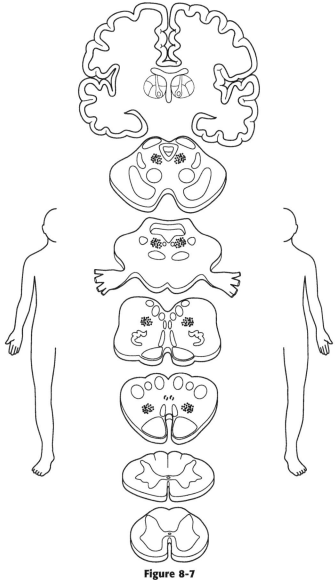

Figure 8-7

Lateral Reticulospinal Pathway

1. Draw the pathway from cortex to body of Figure 8-8.

2. State the function.

3. State where the pathway crosses.

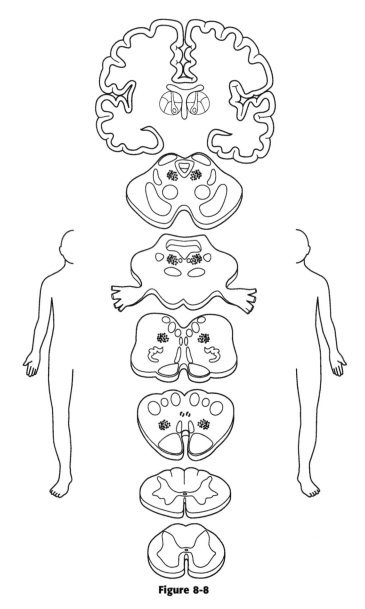

Figure 8-8

Rubrospinal Pathway

1. Draw the pathway from cortex to body on Figure 8-9.

2. State the function.

3. State where the pathway crosses.

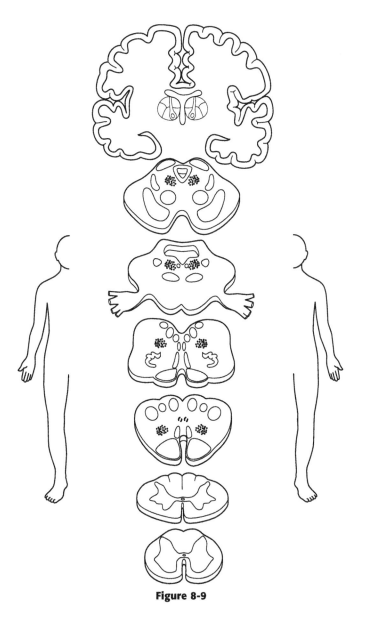

Figure 8-9

Motor System Worksheet

1. The decision to voluntarily move your arm, leg, or body begins in the (identify the lobe) _____.

2. Lower motor neurons have their cell bodies in the _____ of the spinal cord or _____ of the

   brainstem, and travel to the _____ muscle or the muscles of the _____,

   _____, and _____. (Hint: muscles include those of the body and head.)

3. The upper motor neuron cell bodies that begin the voluntary movement pathways originate in the _____.

4. What are the signs of an upper motor neuron lesion?

5. What are the signs of a lower motor neuron lesion?

6. The tectospinal tract begins in the:

7. The vestibulospinal tract begins in the:

8. Which motor pathway is the *most* directly used during functional activities such as tying shoes?

9. The lateral corticospinal tract travels in the _____ of the medulla and the fibers cross in the

   _____.

10. Parker is a 68-year-old male who sustained a right frontal lobe CVA. The primary motor cortex was involved, affecting leg and arm movements. Using the lateral corticospinal tract as your primary motor pathway to understand the symptoms, would Parker demonstrate ipsilateral, contralateral, or bilateral motor symptoms? (Hint: It might help to draw the pathway or refer to your drawings.)

11. Bonnie and Patten were playing on the merry-go-round. The merry-go-round was going very fast and unfortunately Bonnie slipped off and sustained a complete spinal cord injury at L1. Complete the following chart. (Hint: It might help to draw the pathway.)

Pathway	Location	Loss Vs. Intact		Bilateral, Ipsilateral, Contralateral
Lateral corticospinal tract	At the level	Right		
		Left		
	Below the level	Right		
		Left		

Spinal Cord Injury:
Case Stories

Spinal Cord Injury: Case Stories

GOAL

The goal of this lab is for students to use their knowledge of sensory and motor pathways to solve case stories that depict spinal level injuries.

PREPARATION FOR LAB

1. Review sensory and motor pathway drawings, paying particular attention to the location of the pathways in the spinal cord, where the pathway crosses, and the function of the pathway.

2. Complete the lab review of Labs 7 and 8 in preparation for Lab 9.

3. Complete Case Stories 1-5 before the lab.

4. Bring pathway drawings to class to help answer spinal cord case stories 6-8.

5. Additional case stories (9-11) are provided for further practice.

Your lab instructor will check that you have prepared for the lab and will sign below.

_____

Signature of Lab Instructor

REVIEW OF LABS 7 AND 8

Pathways	Function	Crosses at What Level	Note whether the symptoms are ipsilateral or contralateral to the lesion for a lesion in the cortex or brainstem (above the low medulla.)
Are the pathways listed below sensory or motor?			
Spinothalamic			
DCML			
Are the pathways listed below sensory or motor?			
Corticospinal			
Corticobulbar			

CASE STORIES 1-5

Directions: Answer the questions related to each of the following case stories. It is helpful to draw a spinal cord cross section and shade in potential areas of lesion symptoms. This is helpful in determining the actual location of the lesion.

Case No. 1

Samuel and Kool were in a gang fight. Samuel sustained a knife wound in the back that resulted in a hemisection of the first thoracic spinal cord segment on the left side. What signs and symptoms would Samuel experience a few weeks after the initial injury (after the swelling and initial shock of injury have subsided) on the right and left side, at the level of the injury, and below the level of the injury?

Draw a spinal cord cross section of Samuel's injury here:

Sensory and Motor Functions				
			Intact or Loss	**Are the Symptoms: Ipsilateral, Contralateral, Bilateral**
DCML	At level	Right		
		Left		
	Below level	Right		
		Left		
Spinothalamic	At level	Right		
		Left		
	Below level	Right		
		Left		
Lateral corticospinal	At level	Right		
		Left		
	Below level	Right		
		Left		

Case No. 2

Derek and George were hiking Half Dome when an electrical storm blew up. They neglected to heed the warning to turn back and instead hiked to the top. Lightning struck nearby, and they were hit by a falling tree. Derek's lower body was crushed and paralyzed, as he sustained a fracture-dislocation severing the cord at the level of T9-T12. Consequently, he lost movement and sensation in the lower half of his body. What sensory and motor symptoms would Derek demonstrate?

Draw a spinal cord cross section of Derek's injury here:

Sensory and Motor Functions			Intact or Loss	Are the Symptoms: Ipsilateral, Contralateral, Bilateral
DCML	At level	Right		
		Left		
	Below level	Right		
		Left		
Spinothalamic	At level	Right		
		Left		
	Below level	Right		
		Left		
Lateral corticospinal	At level	Right		
		Left		
	Below level	Right		
		Left		

1. What sensations would be lost on the left and right side of his body?

2. Describe the muscular activity at and below the level of the lesion.

3. Would bowel and bladder control be affected? Why or why not?

4. Would sexual function be affected? Why or why not?

Case No. 3

Melanie is a 26-year-old accountant who has recently been hospitalized as a result of some neurological symptoms. You are assigned to her case as her therapist. Her chart indicates that she has a spinal tumor that is being closely watched to determine if it is increasing in size or stabilizing. Her symptoms are predominantly loss of pain and temperature sensation on the left lower extremity and spastic paralysis of the right lower extremity. In addition, some atrophy in the right quadriceps muscles is evident.

Sensory and Motor Functions			Intact or Loss	Are the Symptoms: Ipsilateral, Contralateral, Bilateral
DCML	At level	Right		
		Left		
	Below level	Right		
		Left		
Spinothalamic	At level	Right		
		Left		
	Below level	Right		
		Left		
Lateral corticospinal	At level	Right		
		Left		
	Below level	Right		
		Left		

1. Based on these symptoms, at what level of the spinal cord is the tumor located?

2. Which spinal cord tracts are affected?

3. What is the approximate level of the tumor?

Case No. 4

Terry is a physical therapist who began to notice that she was becoming fatigued more easily during work. She also had experienced decreased muscle power in her upper extremities. Neurological examination revealed bilateral weakness and atrophy in the intrinsic hand muscles and proximal upper extremity musculature, and impaired pain and temperature sensation over most of the right and left upper forearms. All other sensations and motor functions were intact.

Make your own sensory and motor pathway grid to solve this case.

1. Where is the lesion located?

2. What is the extent of the lesion?

3. To what type of lesion are these signs and symptoms most likely due?

Case No. 5

Joshua is a 5-year-old boy who began complaining of a headache. His father took him to the pediatrician two days later because Joshua also had developed a fever and complained of pain in his back and left leg. Upon examination, it was noted that Joshua exhibited flaccid paralysis in his left lower extremity, with beginning atrophy in this area. His deep tendon reflexes were decreased, but his sensations were intact.

Sensory and Motor Functions				
			Intact or Loss	**Are the Symptoms: Ipsilateral, Contralateral, Bilateral**
DCML	At level	Right		
		Left		
	Below level	Right		
		Left		
Spinothalamic	At level	Right		
		Left		
	Below level	Right		
		Left		
Lateral corticospinal	At level	Right		
		Left		
	Below level	Right		
		Left		

1. What area of the spinal cord is affected?

2. What disease most likely caused Joshua's symptoms?

3. What is the approximate level of the lesion, and on which side is it located?

4. Draw a diagram to demonstrate the lesion.

CASE STORIES 6-8

Once you have checked your answers with your lab group for cases 1-5, complete case stories 6-8 in small groups. It is helpful to reference a dermatome chart while you solve these cases, and to keep in mind the difference in symptoms between peripheral and central nervous system injuries.

Case No. 6

David is a 30-year-old pipe fitter. While welding a fitting, he noticed that sparks from the flame landed on his right thumb, but he did not feel any pain. Later he discovered that he had slight burns to the area. He also realized that he had lost some of the muscle power in his right hand and was having some difficulty holding his welding torch. He went to the job-site nurse, who noted anesthesia on his right arm with mild atrophy and decreased strength. All other sensory and motor functions were intact. David told the nurse he had been involved in a car accident a few days before, but was not injured. The RN recommended that he see his physician and a neurologist immediately.

1. David's symptoms are indicative of what type of a neurological dysfunction (peripheral or central)? Why?

2. What are these symptoms most likely due to?

3. What level(s) of the spinal area is (are) affected?

4. What might cause this type of disorder?

5. Draw the location of the lesion in a spinal cord cross section.

Case No. 7

Joe is a 27-year-old policeman. He was called to check a robbery in progress and surprised the robber, who shot Joe in the back. He was admitted to the hospital, and upon neurological examination, he presented the following symptoms: flaccid paralysis at the level of C7-T2 on the left side, spastic musculature from T2 down on the left side, loss of pain and temperature sensation on the right side from about C8 down, loss of position and vibration sense, and loss of tactile sensation on the left side from C7 down.

1. What are the probable type, extent, and level of Joe's lesion?

2. Which muscles would show flaccid paralysis?

3. What symptom related to the spinothalamic tract would be observed at the level of the lesion (C7)? Would these symptoms be bilateral, ipsilateral, or contralateral at C7?

4. Why are pain and temperature sensations lost at C8 and down, while other sensations are lost from C7 down?

Case No. 8

Tom is a 63-year-old male who has been in good health. Recently he noticed increasing difficulty walking and urinating. Often his feet would bounce uncontrollably when he would sit down to watch TV or eat a meal. Upon examination, his physician found mild atrophy in the trunk internal and external oblique muscles bilaterally, spasticity in both lower extremities, and only reflex control of the bladder. Pain and temperature sensations were absent in the lower abdominal area and in both lower extremities; all other sensations were intact.

1. What is the location and extent of Tom's lesion?

2. What type of lesion most likely caused these symptoms?

3. Why is there flaccidity in the obliques and spasticity below that?

4. Why is there involvement in bladder control?

ADDITIONAL CASE STORIES – complete these case stories for additional practice

Case No. 9

Bill is a well-known musician who was recently in a serious auto accident while attempting to round Dead Man's Curve on Kelly Drive. He hit a tree and was pinned between the steering wheel and the car seat. This impact fractured his lower spine. Two months after his accident, he is scheduled for occupational and physical therapy. His chart indicates that he is severely depressed about losing the function of both lower extremities and having to use a catheter. He believes he will no longer be able to function sexually. Neurological examination reveals flaccidity in the majority of both lower extremities, with some intermittent spasticity in the foot musculature. All sensations are impaired in both lower extremities, but are intact in the abdominal and groin area.

1. What is the extent and level of Bill's lesion?

2. What type of bladder and sexual functioning may Bill be capable of, and why?

3. Draw the location of the lesion.

Case No. 10

Jimmy is a 4-year-old child who was born with a lumbar area meningomyelocele. This was surgically repaired during infancy, but has left Jimmy with sensory and motor impairment in both lower extremities. Jimmy presently ambulates with long leg braces and a walker. He is now in a preschool classroom and is referred for OT and PT. Upon evaluation, you note that Jimmy has trace hip flexion and hip extension, and intact sensation in both anterior thigh areas. He does not respond to pain and temperature, tactile sensation, or two-point discrimination on the posterior aspects of both thighs, nor does he respond to these sensations on the lower leg area of both lower extremities. Motorically, Jimmy is able to initiate small amounts of hip flexion and extension without his braces on, but he is unable to move any other parts of his lower extremities. His sensation and motor abilities are intact in his trunk and upper extremities.

1. What is a meningomyelocele?

2. How does it affect the sensory and motor functions in the spinal cord?

3. Based on Jimmy's sensory and motor functions, at what level is his meningomyelocele located? (Hint: Use dermatome and segmental innervations.)

Case No. 11

Jeff is a 35-year-old male. He is an economist by occupation and enjoys long distance running in his free time. During his last marathon, Jeff began to experience some shooting pain down the posterior aspect of his left lower extremity. Like most marathon runners, Jeff chose to ignore this pain. Even after his marathon, Jeff continued running and training at his usual pace, although this pain was becoming worse, until he was unable to get out of bed one morning. He had excruciating pain in his lower back and left leg. Jeff went to the sports medicine center, where it was discovered that the strength in his lower left extremity was decreased and his responses to sensation were diminished.

1. What type of injury does Jeff most likely have?

2. Based on these symptoms, where is this injury most likely located?

10

Vestibular System

Vestibular System

GOAL

The goal of this lab is for students to understand and identify structures that are associated with the vestibular system, understand how vestibular sensations impact function, and understand the relationship between vestibular and visual systems. Lastly, students will be able to identify common symptoms associated with vestibular dysfunction.

PREPARATION FOR LAB

1. Before the lab, complete the questions 1-5 and 7-10 located in this lab section. Please reference your findings with page numbers from a text. This will help you complete the lab in a timely fashion.

Your lab instructor will check that you have prepared for the lab and will sign below.

_____

Signature of Lab Instructor

LAB 10

Vestibular System

1. Using your textbook as a reference, locate the following structures of the labyrinths. In class, look at the model of the labyrinths and locate these structures:

   a. Superior semicircular canal

   b. Horizontal semicircular canals

   c. Posterior semicircular canal

   d. Utricle and saccule

   e. Ampulla of each semicircular canal (SCC)

   f. Vestibulocochlear nerve

2. Label the structures identified on Figure 10-1.

   A. _____

   B. _____

   C. _____

   D. _____

   E. _____

   F. _____

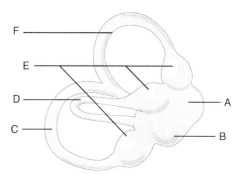

Figure 10-1 Vestibular apparatus.

3. What is the ampulla?

4. Label the structures identified on Figure 10-2.

   A. _____

   B. _____

   C. _____

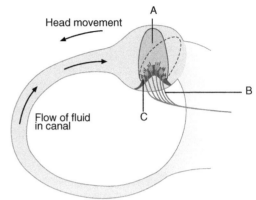

Figure 10-2   The ampulla.

5. What are the stimuli for the SCCs?

6. Nystagmus: Test of the vestibulo-ocular reflex

   Use the postrotary nystagmus board or anchor the base of a rotating chair. Test to be sure the chair will not slip. Have a classmate sit upright and cross-legged in the chair, flex neck forward 30 degrees. Rotate the person clockwise in this position 10 times in 20 seconds. Stop the chair and have your classmate look straight ahead at a blank wall while you observe his or her eye movements.

   Record the length of time of postrotary nystagmus and motion of eyes: horizontal or vertical, and direction of quick versus direction of slow movement of eyes. Outline the events of nystagmus beginning, during, and after rotation.

   A. Beginning rotation to left:

   B. During rotation to left:

   C. After rotation to left:

7. Draw a cross section of the utricle and the saccule, including the otoliths, the macula, and the hair cells. How does the function of the otolith organs differ from the SCC?

8. What are the stimuli for the utricle and saccule?

9. Explain anatomically and physiologically how the utricle, saccule, and semicircular canals detect head movement and position during the lateral labyrinthine righting reaction and other righting and equilibrium reactions.

10. What are the functions of the vestibular system?

11. One of the features of the vestibular system is that it influences movement.

   Refer to Lundy-Ekman (2008) Figures 15-3 and 15-5, pp. 399-400 to help you complete the following drawings. Sketch a brainstem in the space provided below. On the brainstem:

   a. Draw how the vestibular information influences cranial nerve nuclei III, IV, and VI, which impacts extraocular movement.

   b. Draw how the vestibular information influences the muscle activity via the lateral and medial vestibulospinal pathways.

   c. Show how the cerebellum receives information from the vestibular system and modifies it before releasing output information through the superior cerebral peduncle.

Visual System

Visual System

GOAL

The goal of this lab is for students to understand and identify structures that are associated with the visual pathway. Students will also be able to identify common symptoms associated with unilateral and bilateral lesions of the visual pathway.

PREPARATION FOR LAB

1. Before the lecture or lab, read Chapter 15 *Vestibular and Visual Systems* in Lundy-Ekman (2007).

Additional case stories for further practice are found on the Student Evolve Resources.

LAB 11

Vision

1. Draw the pathway of the visual impulse through the lens, retina, optic nerves, optic chiasm, optic tracts, geniculate bodies, and occipital lobes. Pay particular attention to left and right visual fields and how these travel through the optic pathways. *Use colored pencils to identify left temporal, left nasal, right nasal, and right temporal visual fields.*

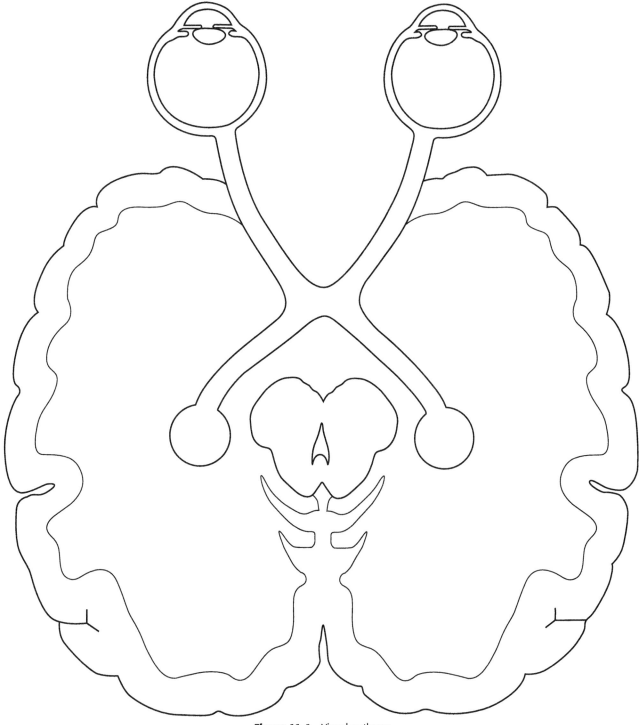

Figure 11-1 Visual pathway

Explain what symptoms will result with a lesion in the following visual areas. Include rationale.

Location of the Lesion	Symptoms
Left optic nerve	
Optic chiasm	
Left optic tract	
Left occipital lobe	

CASE STORY

Sanders is a 63-year-old man who has a significant past medical history including Type II diabetes, arthrosclerosis, arthritis, hypertension, and a right total knee replacement in 2001. Sanders is admitted to the hospital because he was complaining of an excrutiating headache and a change in vision. The MRI revealed that he had a lesion in the right occipital lobe.

a. Using Fig. 11-1, identify the pathways of the visual system that are causing his visual symptoms. What is the term for this symptom?

b. Explain the neurophysiological rationale for the symptom.

Brainstem and Cranial Nerve Case Stories

Brainstem and Cranial Nerve Case Stories

GOAL

The goal of this lab is for students to extend their knowledge about pathways into the brainstem. Students will review the internal and external structures of the brainstem including cranial nerve nuclei, and then solve case stories that demonstrate brainstem or cranial nerve dysfunction.

PREPARATION FOR LAB

1. Complete questive 1-6.

2. Identify the location of the lesion in cases 1-4.

3. Review function of cranial nerves from Lab 4.

Your lab instructor will check that you have prepared for the lab and will sign below.

Signature of Lab Instructor

LAB 12

Questions

Circle the correct answer for question 1:

1. A unilateral lesion in the brainstem often causes loss of function of one or more of the cranial nerves (nuclei). Given the anatomical arrangement of the cranial nerves and nuclei, cranial nerve symptoms would present on the (same or opposite) side as the lesion. In contrast, the person who presents with hemiplegia, sensory and motor loss in the body presents on the (same or opposite) side of the lesion.

2. A lesion involving the oculomotor cranial nucleus would occur at what level of the brainstem?

3. A lesion involving the hypoglossal cranial nucleus would occur at what level of the brainstem?

4. A lesion involving the abducens cranial nucleus would occur at what level of the brainstem?

5. In addition to the cranial nerves, the brainstem also contains the reticular formation. The reticular formation contains

   components important for _____, _____, and _____.

6. Brainstem lesions can result from diverse types of injuries to the central nervous system including:

Brainstem

1. Label the cross sections of the brainstem in Figure 12-1.

BS level _____

A. _____

B. _____

C. _____

D. _____

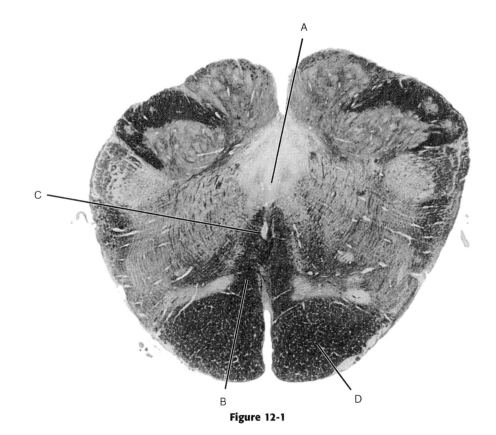

Figure 12-1

2. Label the cross sections of the brainstem in Figure 12-2.

BS level _____

A. _____

B. _____

C. _____

D. _____

E. _____

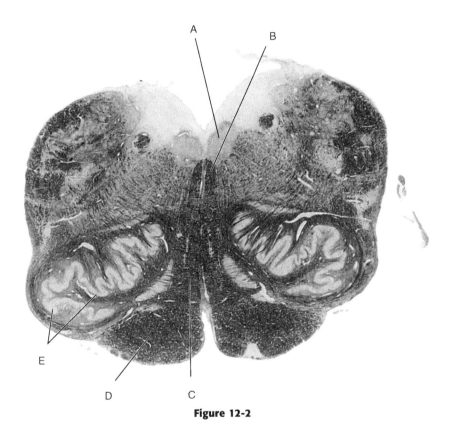

Figure 12-2

3. Label the cross sections of the brainstem in Figure 12-3.

BS level _____

A. _____

B. _____

C. _____

D. _____

E. _____

F. _____

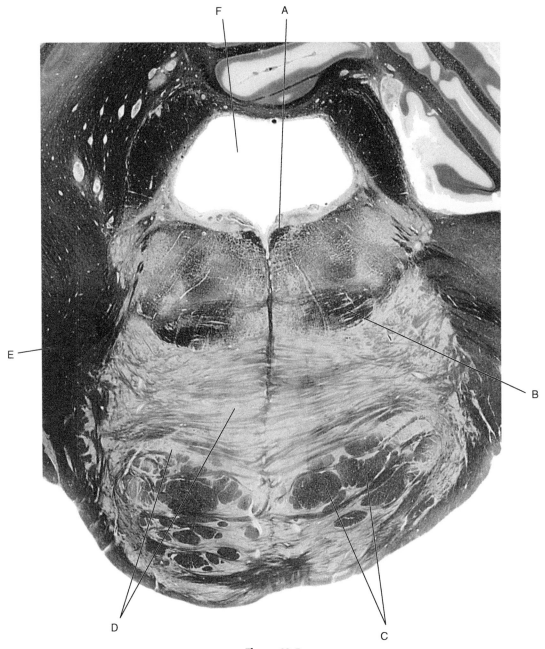

Figure 12-3

4. Label the cross sections of the brainstem in Figure 12-4.

BS level _____

A. _____

B. _____

C. _____

D. _____

E. _____

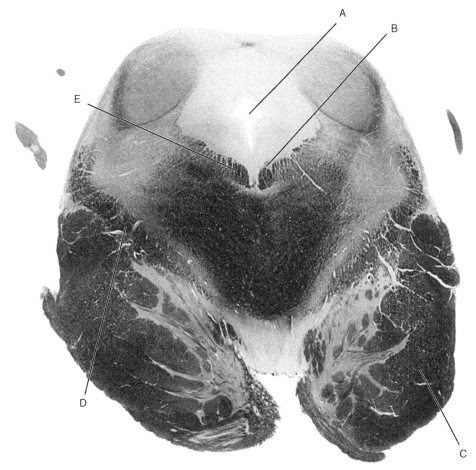

Figure 12-4

5. Label the cross sections of the brainstem in Figure 12-5.

BS level _____

A. _____

B. _____

C. _____

D. _____

E. _____

F. _____

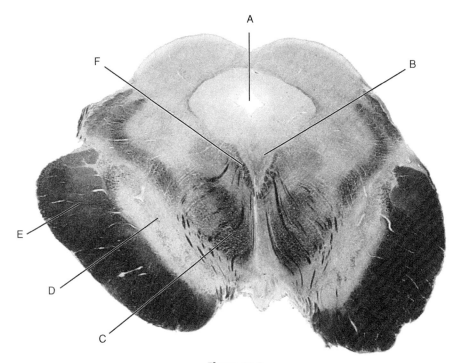

Figure 12-5

CASE STORIES 1-4

Directions: For each case story, list the anatomical structure affected and the rationale for each symptom.

CASE NO. 1

Signs and Symptoms	Anatomical Structure and Rationale
Flaccid paralysis of all muscles of facial expression on the right side	
Some loss of conscious proprioception on the left side of the body	
Internal strabismus of the right eye	

1. Draw a cross section of the lesion.

2. The lesion is located in what part of the brainstem? How do you know it is a brainstem lesion?

3. A lesion of what artery or arteries might cause these symptoms?

CASE NO. 2

Signs and Symptoms	Anatomical Structure and Rationale
Anesthetic on the left side of the face	
Muscles of mastication are paralyzed and atrophied on the left	
Tongue points to the left when protruded	
Spastic type of hemiplegia in the right trunk and limbs on the right	

1. Draw a cross section of the lesion.

2. The lesion is located in what part of the brainstem? How do you know it is a brainstem lesion?

3. A lesion of what artery or arteries might cause these symptoms?

CASE NO. 3

Signs and Symptoms	Anatomical Structure and Rationale
Spastic paralysis and/or hemiplegia on the left side with involvement of arm and leg	
External strabismus of right eye, ptosis of right upper eyelid, dilation of right pupil, loss of the ability to raise the right upper eyelid, loss of movement of the eye	

1. Draw a cross section of the lesion.

2. The lesion is located in what part of the brainstem? How do you know it is a brainstem lesion?

3. A lesion of what artery or arteries might cause these symptoms?

CASE NO. 4

Signs and Symptoms	Anatomical Structure and Rationale
Diminished hearing ipsilateral on the right side	
Decreased balance and vertigo	
Loss of facial expression on the right	
Paralysis of right side of face	

1. Draw a cross section of the lesion.

2. The lesion is located in what part of the brainstem? How do you know it is a brainstem lesion?

3. A lesion of what artery or arteries might cause these symptoms?

Brainstem, Cranial Nerve, and Cerebral Lesions Case Stories

Brainstem, Cranial Nerve, and Cerebral Lesions Case Stories

GOAL

The goal of this lab is for students to solve case stories that illustrate brainstem, cranial nerve, and cerebral dysfunction.

PREPARATION FOR LAB

1. Complete case stories 1-6. Please reference your findings with page numbers from a neuroscience text. Bring these case stories to lab and review them with your lab group to determine if you all obtained the same answer. Discuss your findings. Next, complete case stories 7-10 with your lab group.
2. Additional case studies (11-13) are provided for further practice.

Your lab instructor will check that you have prepared for the lab and will sign below.

_____

Signature of Lab Instructor

CASE STORIES 1-6

Complete the following case stories prior to lab.

Case No. 1

A 23-year-old woman lost her vision in her left eye and then partly recovered it. A diagnosis of multiple sclerosis was suspected but not established. She suffered another attack in a different part of the nervous system three years later. After this second attack, the neurological findings were: (a) spastic weakness and increased reflexes in the right arm and leg with a Babinski sign in the right foot; (b) loss of vibration and position sense in the right arm and leg; (c) internal strabismus of the left eye (left eye turned inward when the right eye is looking forward); and (d) flaccid paralysis of the whole left side of the face, including the forehead.

1. The first two findings above result from a lesion of the sensory and motor tracts, respectively the _____

   and _____. Both are affected on the _____ side of the brain.

2. The last two findings above indicate the level of the lesion. The level is the _____on the

   _____ side.

Circle the correct answer:

3. The spastic paralysis of the arm and leg results from a lesion of the (upper or lower) motor neurons. The flaccid paralysis results from a lesion of (upper or lower) motor neurons.

Case No. 2

1. A lesion in the left corticospinal tract in the upper medulla causes spastic paralysis of the arm and leg on the _____

   _____ (ipsilateral or contralateral) side. A lesion in the left lower medulla (inferior to the decussation) in the left

   pyramidal tract causes spastic paralysis of arm and leg on the _____ (ipsilateral or contralateral) side?

   (Hint: Draw a picture of the medulla. Note where the pyramidal tract crosses the midline.)

Case No. 3

A 7-year-old child was referred to occupational therapy (OT) because he was having difficulty with his schoolwork. Upon evaluation, the occupational therapist noted the child had difficulty expressing himself verbally and used his left hand for all fine motor tasks, even though there was no familial tendency for left-handedness. His attempts at fine motor activities with his right upper extremity were uncoordinated. He demonstrated some incoordination, particularly with activities that required the use of both sides of the body together, such as riding a tricycle or swinging on swings. The neurological report indicated no focal neurological signs, and a CAT scan indicated no visible brain lesion.

1. Based on the above symptoms, what is the most likely location of the lesion? What is the most likely type of lesion? (Hint: right or left hemisphere)

Case No. 4

A 3-year-old girl is referred to OT and PT. She demonstrates increased tone and spastic paralysis of both lower extremities, with minimal involvement of both upper extremities. She demonstrates decreased sensory awareness of both lower extremities and evidence of primitive reflexes in her lower extremities (i.e., positive supporting, flexor withdrawal). Her language, cognition, and problem solving skills appear age appropriate.

1. Based on the above symptoms, what is the most likely location of the lesion? (Hint: think homunculus)

2. To what type of dysfunction are these symptoms most likely related?

Case No. 5

A 72-year-old male arrived in the clinic with the following signs and symptoms: "pill-rolling" tremors in both upper extremities, which decrease when purposeful movement is attempted. He is unable to rise from a sitting position without assistance. When ambulating, he has difficulty stopping, and he shuffles his feet. Rigidity is noted, most marked in the upper extremities. His facial expression appears masklike.

1. These symptoms are most likely due to what disease?

2. Explain the anatomical structures and rationale for each of these symptoms.

Case No. 6

A 9-year-old girl is referred to OT because she is having difficulty reading and writing in school. She often reverses her letters when copying off the blackboard. She has difficulty spatially orienting and navigating herself around the environment and often "gets lost" in school. However, with verbal directions, she can find her way back to the classroom very well. The teacher also noted that she demonstrates some fine motor incoordination. The teacher recommended an OT evaluation and, upon evaluation, the therapist notes difficulty with spatial perceptions of letters and position in space. She has decreased tactile responses of the left upper and lower extremities and prefers to use her right hand (almost exclusively) for fine motor tasks, even during activities that prompt the use of both upper extremities.

1. Based on the above description, what brain area(s) may be contributing to this child's difficulties? (Hint: left or right hemisphere)

CASE STORIES 7-10

Case No. 7

A 63-year-old construction worker was admitted to an acute rehab setting to receive OT and PT. The occupational therapist evaluated him in the morning as part of his dressing routine. The therapist noted that the patient had difficulty dressing and failed to shave the left side of his face. He had difficulty drawing or copying shapes. His left upper and lower extremities were often hanging off the wheelchair, and when repositioned by the therapist, they frequently slid off again with no apparent recognition of these occurrences by the patient. Sensory testing indicated decreased sensory awareness of the left upper and lower extremities. Motor testing revealed weakness in both left lower and upper extremities. The OT informed the PT of the evaluation results.

1. Based on the above symptoms, what is the most likely location of the lesion? To what type of lesion might this condition be due?

Case No. 8

A 40-year-old female was referred for an OT/PT evaluation in an outpatient setting. She demonstrated constant irregular movements of her body, along with facial grimacing and lip smacking. There was no spastic paralysis. She walked with a dancelike or lurching gait.

1. These symptoms are most likely due to what disease?

2. Outline the anatomical structures and rationale for each of these symptoms.

Case No. 9

A 35-year-old woman was referred to OT/PT for evaluation. The therapist noted that the woman had some difficulty walking because her gait was wide-based and uncoordinated, and she often veered to the left. There was an intention tremor present in the left upper and lower extremities. Past-pointing also was noted. Diadochokinesia of the left upper extremity was deficient.

1. Identify the lesion in the above case and give the anatomical rationale for each symptom.

Case No. 10

The cerebellopontine angle is a common site for tumor development and pressure involvement, related to the cranial nerves in this area.

1. What is the cerebellopontine angle? Where is it? What cranial nerves are in this area? What symptoms might you anticipate after an injury to this area?

ADDITIONAL CASE STORIES

The following case stories are for additional practice and can be completed in lab if time permits or used for additional practice.

Case No. 11

A 70-year-old male was brought into the emergency room on Thursday night, admitted to the hospital immediately, and referred to OT and PT two days later. Upon admission to the ER, his symptoms included external strabismus of the right eye, paresis of the left upper and lower limbs, hypertonicity and hyperreflexia of both limbs on the left side, and Babinski sign on the left.

1. Based on these symptoms, what is the likely location of the lesion?

Case No. 12

A 50-year-old truck driver was brought to the hospital, unconscious after he collapsed while loading his truck. After he regained consciousness, an examination revealed the following symptoms: hypertonicity and spastic paralysis of both right extremities, with increased deep tendon reflexes; deviation of the tongue to the left when protruded; dysarthria; and loss of position sense, pressure, and two-point discriminative touch on the right side.

1. Based on these symptoms, what is the likely location of the lesion? To what type of lesion might this be due?

ADDITIONAL INFORMATION AND CLARIFICATION ABOUT TONGUE INNERVATION AND MOVEMENT

A lower motor neuron lesion of cranial nerve or nuclei XII results in tongue deviation toward the side of lesion due to atrophy on *same* side (see Lundy-Ekman p. 371, Table 13-4 and Nolte, 2008, p. 304)

EXAMPLE: lesion in the *right* nuclei of CN XII → tongue deviates to *right* side b/c muscle atrophy on the *right*

When there is a UMN lesion there is a loss of inhibition on the contralateral nuclei. This creates increased tone and the tongue deviates to the opposite side.

The cranial nerve that innervates the tongue is the hypoglossal nerve. The hypoglossal nucleus is a thin structure that forms an elevation known as the hypoglossal trigone or triangle in the rostral and caudal medulla. Information from this nucleus travels ipsilaterally through fibers that exit between the pyramids and inferior olive. The fibers (hypoglossal nerve) innervate the tongue ipsilaterally (Nolte, 2008, p. 304).

The tongue consists of two primary muscles that oppose each other. When a person is asked to stick out their tongue both muscles contract against each other allowing the tongue to move forward.

If a lesion affects the hypoglossal nucleus or nerve, the muscles of the tongue on the same side become weak and eventually atrophy. The tongue deviates to the same side as the lesion (toward the weaker side) (Nolte, 2008, p. 304).

CASE NO. 13

Marcutio wanted to become a doctor at a very young age. He survived brain cancer and was inspired to save others. He is currently in a residency program at a large city hospital. For several weeks Marcutio has been complaining of headaches, but has been ignoring them, thinking they are related to his job and lack of sleep. One morning after he wakes up, he goes to the bathroom to wash his face and brush his teeth. When he dries his face he notices that his tongue is pointing to the left in the mirror. He quickly retracts his tongue, and then slowly sticks it out again, noticing his tongue moves to the left.

If we assume Marcutio's cancer may have returned, and it is a lower motor neuron lesion, on which side of the brainstem would the lesion be located?

14

Student Teaching
Assignment

Student Teaching Assignment

Each student will teach about a chosen lesion to fellow classmates in their lab group. The student will present a case story in which signs and symptoms of a particular disorder are illustrated. Then, fellow classmates will identify where the lesion is, based on the symptoms. The student will then draw the lesion for their classmates to demonstrate the location of the lesion.

Students will randomly select their lesion from an envelope containing the following areas (note that an area may be represented more than one time, depending on the number of students):

- Spinal cord
- Brainstem (including reticular formation and vestibular system)
- Peripheral nervous system
- Muscle spindle/GTO
- Cerebellum
- Cortex: frontal, parietal, occipital, temporal
- Basal ganglion and related areas
- Cerebellum
- Limbic system
- Special senses

Note to Instructor: Instructor should record which student is teaching the specific lesion. Students should be encouraged NOT to share case stories.

Other lesions may be approved by instructors. The lesion should be one that has been discussed or covered in class.

CRITERIA FOR STUDENT TEACHING ASSIGNMENT

Students need to have the following prepared for their presentation:

1. A 3 × 5-inch index card with the name of the lesion on the front of the card
2. Correct list of the signs and symptoms of the lesion on the back of the card
3. List of reliable reference(s) other than the class notes in APA format
4. Presentation:
   a. Correctly draw the lesion on the board
   b. Correctly explain the signs and symptoms related to the lesion
   c. Present signs and symptoms of the lesion (disorder) in a case story

Grading:

A+
Includes all criteria listed above, plus creativity in case story or in presentation

A
Includes all criteria listed above (6 components)

B+
Includes requirements 1, 2, 3, 4a, 4b, or 4c (5 of 6 components), plus creativity in case story or in presentation

B
Includes requirements 1, 2, 3, 4a, 4b, or 4c (5 of 6 components)

B-
Includes 4 of 6 requirements completed correctly

C+
Includes only 3 of 6 requirements completed correctly, plus creativity

C
Includes only 3 of 6 requirements completed correctly

D+
Includes only 2 of 6 requirements completed successfully (No. 2 and 4b = 1 unit), plus creativity

D
Includes only 2 of 6 requirements completed successfully (No. 2 and 4b = 1 unit)

F
Incorrectly lists signs and symptoms on index card, regardless of other components

Figure Credits

CPI Antony Rowe
Eastbourne, UK
August 05, 2019